Principles & Practicalities of Oral & Maxillofacial Surgery

An accessible guide to oral and maxillofacial surgery (OMFS). Written by a renowned group of clinical specialists, it ensures that the principles and the practicalities of OMFS are easily understood by both doctors and dentists at all stages of their training.

Inside, each section includes coverage of

- How to prepare for patients
- Key points in the patient history and examination
- How best to investigate and manage a range of OMFS presentations and conditions

Each chapter is structured to provide an easy reference, including red flag and primary care sections to enable readers to know what to look out for when considering referrals. The inclusion of multiple-choice questions (MCQs) at the end of each chapter helps to test understanding of the chapter material and reinforce learning.

Whether you're approaching medical school finals, MRCS examinations, or higher surgical training in OMFS, *Principles & Practicalities of Oral & Maxillofacial Surgery* is your guide to understanding and navigating the complexities of this demanding specialty.

In the same series

Principles and Practicalities of ENT
Keshav K. Gupta, Divya Vatish, Karan Jolly, Duncan Bowyer

Principles & Practicalities of Oral & Maxillofacial Surgery

How to approach common clinical scenarios

Edited by

Keshav K. Gupta
and Ahmed Abdelrahman

CRC Press
Taylor & Francis Group
Boca Raton New York London

CRC Press is an imprint of the
Taylor & Francis Group, an **informa** business

Designed cover image: Shutterstock

First edition published 2026
by CRC Press
2385 NW Executive Center Drive, Suite 320, Boca Raton FL 33431

and by CRC Press
4 Park Square, Milton Park, Abingdon, Oxon, OX14 4RN

CRC Press is an imprint of Taylor & Francis Group, LLC

ISBN: 9781032796734 (hbk)
ISBN: 9781032803357 (pbk)
ISBN: 9781003493310 (ebk)

DOI: 10.1201/9781003493310

Typeset in LTC Goudy Oldstyle Pro
by Apex CoVantage, LLC

To Ma, for her endless display of love throughout her life.

Keshav K. Gupta

To my beloved wife, Amira, whose unwavering support, love, and encouragement have been my constant source of strength throughout this journey, and to my wonderful daughters, Maryam and Safiya, whose smiles light up my world and whose boundless curiosity inspire me every day. This book is for you, my family – my greatest achievements and my endless motivation.

Ahmed Abdelrahman

Contents

Preface

Principles & Practicalities of Oral & Maxillofacial Surgery (OMFS) is a resource allowing students, dentists and doctors of all levels to approach common clinical scenarios encountered in OMFS with confidence. A companion to *Principles and Practicalities of ENT*, each section will take you through how to prepare for patients and examination, key points in the history and how best to investigate and manage a wide variety of OMFS presentations and conditions. The material is structured to provide an easy reference, including red flag and primary care sections to enable readers to know what to look out for when considering referrals. There are also some multiple-choice questions (MCQs) at the end of each chapter to help solidify understanding of the chapter material and reinforce learning. Therefore, in addition to being a revision tool for medical school finals, MRCS examinations and higher surgical training in OMFS, this book can also serve as a useful everyday aid for physicians in their assessment, diagnostics, management and referral practices. Overall, we hope that this essential guide, combining practical insights and clinical expertise, will be an invaluable resource for trainees and practitioners alike.

Editors

Keshav K. Gupta is an ENT Surgical Specialty Registrar working in the West Midlands in the NHS. He graduated with multiple prizes and distinctions from Imperial College London in 2017. Since then, Gupta has maintained a strong research interest having published more than 45 peer-reviewed articles, multiple book chapters and headed the *Principles and Practicalities of ENT* title published in 2023. In addition, his work has been presented nationally and internationally at numerous surgical conferences where he has won several prizes. Alongside his clinical work, Gupta is also an Associate Editor of the *Clinical Otolaryngology* journal, and a clinical personal academic tutor for medical students at the University of Birmingham.

Ahmed Abdelrahman is a Consultant Oral and Maxillofacial Surgeon specializing in head and neck oncology and reconstruction at University Hospital Coventry and Warwickshire, UK. With a distinguished career spanning over 15 years, Abdelrahman holds dual qualifications in medicine and dentistry, graduating with distinction from Cairo University in 2004 and earning his MBChB from the University of Birmingham in 2014. He completed his surgical training and achieved CCT in 2023. A passionate educator and researcher, Abdelrahman has published more than 20 peer-reviewed articles, with his work presented at national and international conferences. He was awarded the prestigious Norman Rowe Clinical Prize in 2019 for his contributions to the field. He is the founder of the Maxillofacial Audit and Research Collaborative (West Midlands) and is a digital surgical teaching fellow, actively involved in developing innovative educational programs such as the West Midlands Microvascular Simulation Course.

Contributors

Ms Zahra Al Asaadi BDS BSc MBChB MFDS MRCS
Specialty OMFS Registrar
Wessex Deanery, UK

Dr Sherif Amer BDS MSc
Speciality Doctor
University Hospitals Coventry and Warwickshire, UK

Mr Adil Aslam BDS (Hons) MBChB (Hons) MRCS FRCS (OMFS)
OMFS Consultant
Worcestershire Acute Hospitals NHS Trust, UK

Mr William Breakey MBBS BSc (Hons) PhD FRCS (Plast)
Cleft and Plastic Surgery Consultant
Leeds Teaching Hospital Trust & Yorkshire Cleft Service, UK

Lieutenant Colonel John Breeze FRCS FDS PhD
OMFS Consultant
University Hospitals Birmingham, UK

Dr Clayton Davis DDS, MD, MSc, FRCD(C)
Associate Professor, OMFS Surgeon
University of Alberta, Canada

Mr Shofiq Islam MBBCh BDS MFDSRCS DOHNS FRCS MD
OMFS Consultant
University Hospitals Coventry and Warwickshire, UK

Mr Ashwin Kerai BDS (Hons) MFDS RCSEd MBChB FRCS (OMFS)
TIG Mohs Micrographic Surgery Fellow
Whiston Hospital, UK

Mr Farhan Khalid BDS MFDS FFD MBChB PGCert (Teaching) PGCert (OMFS) FRCS (OMFS)
OMFS Consultant
Bradford Teaching Hospitals, UK

Mr David McGoldrick BDS MBBCh MSc FFD RCSI (OSOM) FRCS (OMFS)
OMFS Consultant
Mater Misericordiae University Hospital, Ireland

Mr Niall M.H. McLeod BDS MBBCh FRCS (OMFS) FDS
OMFS Consultant
University Hospitals Coventry and Warwickshire, UK

Mr Kevin McMillan BDS MBBS MFDRCSI FRCS (OMFS)
OMFS Consultant
University Hospitals Birmingham, UK

Mr Sat Parmar BChD BMBS BMedSci FDSRCS FRCS FRCS (OMFS)
OMFS Consultant
University Hospitals Birmingham, UK

Mr Prav Praveen BDS MBChB FRCS (OMFS) FDSRCS FFDRCSI
OMFS Consultant
University Hospitals Birmingham, UK

Mr Peter Stockton FRCS (OMFS)
OMFS Consultant
University Hospitals Coventry and Warwickshire, UK

Mr Salman Tahir MBBCh BAO MRCS FFDRCSI FCPS BDS
Speciality OMFS Registrar
West Midlands Deanery, UK

Dr Neha Vatish BDS
General Dental Practitioner
London, UK

Mr Justin Jui Yuan Yeo MBChB MRCS (ENT)
Specialty ENT Surgery Registrar
West Midlands Deanery, UK

Mr Daanesh Zakai BDS (Wales) MFDS MBChB FRCS (OMFS)
TMJ and Orthognathic Surgery Fellow
University of Alberta, Canada

Abbreviations

3D	3-dimensional	FNAC	fine needle aspiration cytology
ABG	alveolar bone graft		
ALS	Advanced Life Support	FNE	flexible nasoendoscopy
ALT	anterolateral thigh	FONA	front of neck access
AMPLE	allergies, medications, past medical history, last meal, events leading to presentation	Fr	French
		g	gram
		GA	general anaesthetic
		GCS	Glasgow Coma Score
		GP	general practitioner
ATLS	Advanced Trauma Life Support	Gy	gray
		Hb	haemoglobin
AV	arteriovenous	HFNC	high-flow nasal cannula
AVM	arteriovenous malformation	HIV	human immunodeficiency virus
BAD	British Association of Dermatologists	HPV	human papillomavirus
		HR	heart rate
BCC	basal cell carcinoma	ICU	intensive care unit
BP	blood pressure	IHD	ischaemic heart disease
cSCC	cutaneous squamous cell carcinoma	ISSVA	International Society for the Study of Vascular Anomalies
cm	centimetre		
CN	cranial nerve	IV	intravenous
CO_2	carbon dioxide	kg	kilogram
COPD	chronic obstructive pulmonary disease	L	litre
		LA	local anaesthetic
CPR	cardiopulmonary resuscitation	LLLT	low-level laser therapy
		LVI	lymphovascular invasion
CRP	C-reactive protein		
CT	computed tomography	MAL	methyl aminolevulinate
CXR	chest x-ray	mc&s	microscopy, sensitivity & culture
DCIA	deep circumflex iliac artery		
		MCQ	multiple-choice question
DOI	depth of invasion	MDT	multidisciplinary team
DPT	dental panoramic topogram	mg	milligram
		MIO	maximum inter-incisal opening
DVT	deep vein thrombosis		
EAC	external auditory canal	ml	millilitres
ECG	electrocardiogram	mm	millimetres
ED	emergency department	MMF	mandibular-maxillary fixation
ENT	ear, nose and throat		
ESWL	extracorporeal shockwave lithotripsy	mmHg	millimeters of mercury
		MRI	magnetic resonance imaging
FAMMM	familial atypical multiple mole melanoma syndrome	MRONJ	medication-related osteonecrosis of the jaw
FBC	full blood count		

NBM	nil by mouth	SCC	squamous cell carcinoma
NG	nasogastric	SLNB	sentinel lymph node
NGT	nasogastric tube		biopsy
NHSP	Newborn Hearing	SLT	speech and language
	Screening Programme		therapy
NSAID	non-steroidal anti-	SOB	shortness of breath
	inflammatory drug	SpO$_2$	oxygen saturation
OMFS	oral maxillofacial surgery	SPECT	single positron emission
OPG	orthopantomogram		computed tomography
ORIF	open reduction internal	SPF	sun protection factor
	fixation	TB	tuberculosis
ORN	osteoradionecrosis	TJR	total joint replacement
PA	posteroanterior	TMD	temporomandibular joint
PDS	polydioxanone suture		disorder
PDT	photodynamic therapy	TMJ	temporomandibular joint
PET	positron emission	TNM	tumour, node, metastasis
	tomography		staging classification
PNI	perineural invasion	U&Es	urea and electrolytes
PVD	peripheral vascular	URTI	upper respiratory tract
	disease		infection
RAPD	relative afferent pupillary	US	ultrasound
	defect	USS	ultrasound scan
RR	respiratory rate	UV	ultraviolet
RTA	road traffic accident	VBG	venous blood gas
s	second	XR	x-ray

Section I

Emergency

Odontogenic infections

Salman Tahir and Peter Stockton

Background

Odontogenic infections are infections of the alveolus, jaw or face originating from an infected tooth or its supporting structures. The most common causes are dental caries, complications of recent dental work (deep fillings, failed root canal treatment) or periodontal disease. In the early phase, patients can experience pain and swelling. If the infection progresses, abscess formation is possible as well as further spread through fascial planes of the head and neck (Figure 1.1) that can contribute to deep neck space infections and added morbidity including airway compromise.

Potential areas for deterioration

A airway compromise secondary to oropharynx / submandibular / sublingual swelling
C septic shock
D cavernous sinus thrombosis can be sight-threatening and risk of intracranial extension

Preparation and equipment

- This is an OMFS emergency and the patient must be seen to promptly.
- Involve members of the MDT early if signs of airway compromise including anaesthetics and ENT.

History

Symptoms – pain, swelling

- Onset, timing and duration
- Laterality
- Better or worse
- Preceding events – dental infection, dental work
- Previous episodes

DOI: 10.1201/9781003493310-2

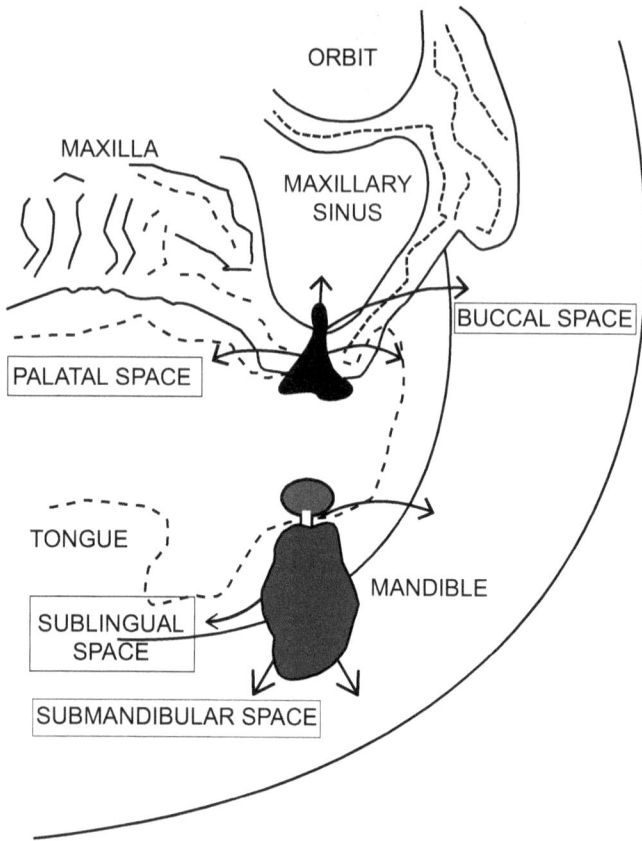

Figure 1.1 Potential areas of spread from maxillary or mandibular dental infections. Maxillary teeth can also lead to cavernous sinus thrombosis via the facial vein to the cavernous sinus. Mandibular tooth infections can spread to the parapharyngeal space and mediastinum. Swelling involving oropharynx can contribute to airway compromise.

Systems

- Airway – SOB, aspiration/choking, drooling
- Oesophagus – rapid onset dysphagia, odynophagia, regurgitation
- Oral cavity – overall dental hygiene and condition
- Voice – rapid onset change in voice

Risk factors/Red flags

- Recent dental infection/treatment
- Smoking, alcohol
- Poor oral/dental hygiene
- Diabetes, immunocompromise

AMPLE

- Allergies, regular/recent medications, other relevant past medical history, time of last meal

Examination

- General inspection for signs of respiratory distress – noisy breathing (stridor, stertor), tachypnoea, cyanosis, use of accessory muscles, anxiety, agitation, fatigue, drooling
- Voice – speaking in full sentences, quality of voice, hoarseness
- Neck – range of motion and torticollis, lumps, cellulitis, swelling
- Oral cavity/oropharynx – tongue and floor of mouth swelling (raised tongue), tonsils, peritonsillar swelling, halitosis, swelling (buccal/palatal), trismus
- Dentition – broken/carous teeth (tender to percussion), infected tooth
- Skin – assess for signs of cellulitis on the overlying skin (Figure 1.2)
- Full set of observations – assess for signs of respiratory distress (tachypnoea, reduced saturations) or sepsis (tachycardia, fever, hypotension)

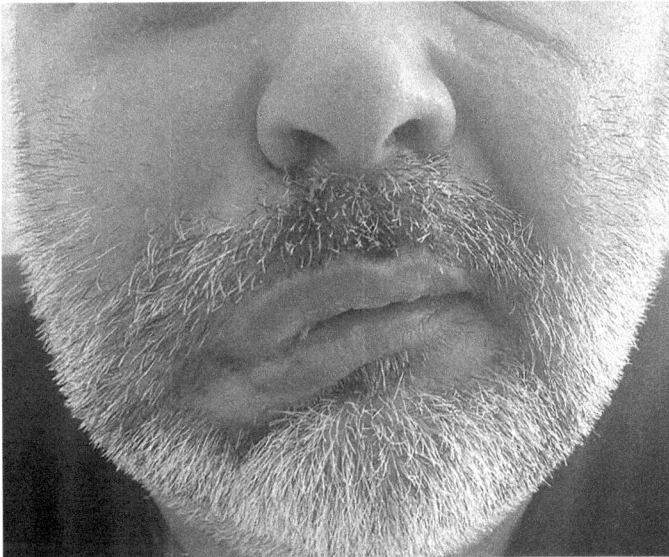

Figure 1.2 Odontogenic infection of the upper-right 6 (UR6) with subsequent right facial swelling, asymmetry, cellulitis and lower eyelid involvement.

Management

The principle of management in patients with odontogenic infection is to treat the infection, remove the source and prevent any complications. The acute infection can often be treated with antibiotics but may require surgical drainage and extraction of the offending tooth. Prompt treatment and intervention is vital to minimise the risk of potentially life-threatening complications. If the patient presents with a critical airway, this should be dealt with as a priority.

Bedside

- Swab – mc&s any discharge in oral cavity
- Bloods – FBC, U&E, CRP, lactate, blood cultures, HbA1c

Imaging

- OPG – dental cause (Figure 1.3) – carous/offending tooth, abscess
- CT neck with contrast (Figure 1.4) – if unable to examine oral cavity, suspicion of deep space neck infection, systemic signs, concerns about swallowing or airway

Localised abscess

- IV antibiotics
- Incision and drainage of abscess (LA)
- Extraction of causative tooth (LA) – same time or semi-elective basis
- Refer back to dentist if tooth is salvageable

Abscess extension/Systemic involvement

- IV antibiotics
- Incision and drainage of abscess + extraction of causative tooth/teeth (GA)
- Neck exploration may be warranted in cases of deep neck space infections

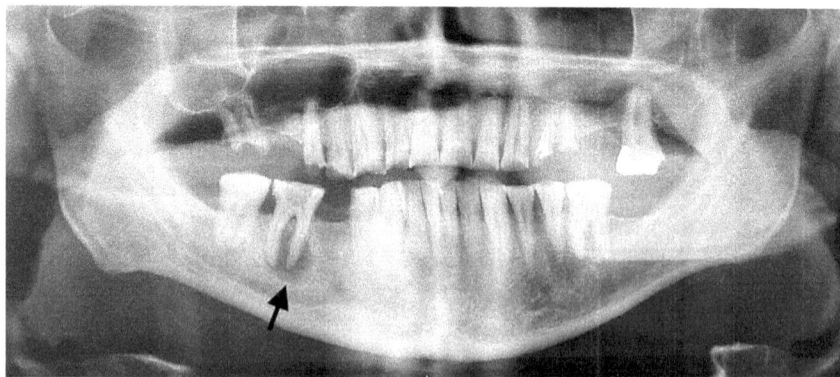

Figure 1.3 **Periapical infection in the right mandibular molar tooth.**

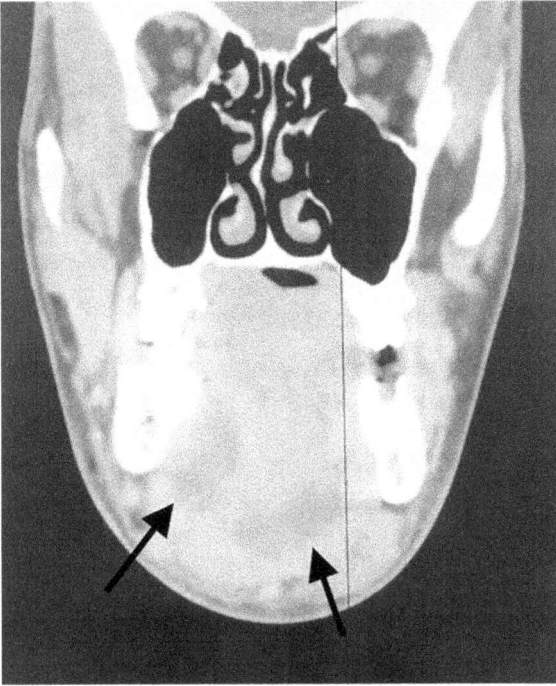

Figure 1.4 Coronal view of CT scan showing spread of collection in right submandibular and submental spaces.

Discharge and follow-up

- Discharge once satisfactory clinical recovery – symptoms, examination, inflammatory markers, all surgical drains removed (if any)
- Repeat imaging is usually not indicated
- Discharge on oral antibiotics, mouthwash and advice regarding strict oral hygiene
- Follow-up is usually in 1–2 weeks depending on the local policy

MCQs

1) A 25-year-old male presents to the emergency department with a 5-day history of progressive swelling in the right submandibular region extending into the neck. He describes some difficulty in swallowing and was getting hot and cold flushes the previous night. He recently visited his dentist for pain in the right mandibular first molar tooth, for which he had the first stage of root canal treatment. He is haemodynamically stable and self-presented to ED. What will be your immediate concern in this patient?

   A) Start IV antibiotics and IV fluids
   B) Bloods and lactate
   C) Airway assessment and management
   D) Drain the infection in ED
   E) Discharge on oral antibiotics

2) A 40-year-old medically fit and well woman presents to ED with pain and swelling in right cheek which started 2 days ago. She went to the dentist with pain in right maxillary canine tooth, for which the dentist started her on oral antibiotics. On examination she has normal vital signs. There is a localised swelling in the right maxillary buccal vestibule adjacent to the right maxillary canine tooth. There is no palatal swelling, normal mouth opening and a soft floor of mouth with mobile tongue. Her WCC is 12 and CRP is 48. What would be the best management for this patient?

   A) Immediate airway management
   B) Admission for IV antibiotic and IV fluids
   C) Incision and drainage of maxillary abscess under LA or GA ± extraction of tooth
   D) Extraoral incision and drainage under LA
   E) Discharge on oral antibiotics

3) A 75-year-old male presents to ED at 11 PM with 6-day history of right neck swelling starting from the right cheek and extending into the right submandibular region. He informs you that he went to the dentist who identified that his last mandibular molar tooth has significant unrestorable caries, but due to limited mouth opening could not carry out the dental extraction. He is vitally stable, apyretic with WCC 16 and CRP 120. He can communicate with you in clear sentences and is able to swallow liquids. His CT scan shows a collection in submandibular space. What is the best management option?

   A) Call anaesthetist for immediate airway assessment
   B) Transfer the patient immediately to theatre for incision and drainage
   C) Admit for IV antibiotics and plan for incision and drainage tomorrow
   D) Extraoral incision and drainage in ED
   E) Discharge patient on oral antibiotic with follow-up in outpatient

Chapter 2

Osteomyelitis

Sherif Amer and Shofiq Islam

Background

Craniofacial osteomyelitis is a rare but serious condition with significant morbidity due to pain, dysfunction and a requirement for a prolonged treatment course. It can present in a variety of ways including pain, erythema, swelling, discharge, evidence of exposed bone or even as a late presentation with more severe complications. It represents a complex clinical condition necessitating timely diagnosis and treatment to prevent detrimental sequelae including sepsis, dental mobility, fistulae (intraoral and extraoral), labiomental numbness, osteonecrosis / pathological fractures and extension to the mouth (oro-antral communication), orbit and intracranial cavity. Osteomyelitis of the mandible usually develops as a result of direct spread from a dentoalveolar infection secondary to a necrotic pulp, inadequate root canal treatment, periodontal disease, fracture or dental extraction. While haematogenous spread is less common as a cause, it can be seen in very young patients. Maxillary osteomyelitis is far less common than mandibular due to the extensive blood circulation, thin cortex and limited medullary tissue in the maxilla. Osteomyelitis can be acute (<1 month) or chronic (>1 month) with chronic further subdivided into suppurative and sclerosing osteomyelitis. Patients under 20 years may present with Garre osteomyelitis in which there is proliferative osteitis on a background of osteomyelitis as a consequence of a long-standing low-grade dentoalveolar infection.

Differential diagnosis

- Neoplastic – intra-bony SCC, multiple myeloma, lymphoma
- Benign – fibro-osseous lesions
- Paediatrics – osteosarcoma, Ewing's sarcoma, fibrous dysplasia

Potential areas for deterioration

C septic shock

Preparation and equipment

- Patients with suspected osteomyelitis should be seen to promptly, which may be in an acute or clinic setting.

DOI: 10.1201/9781003493310-3

History

Symptoms – may be variable

- Onset, timing and duration
- Overlying skin changes
- Better or worse
- Progression
- Preceding factors – e.g., dental infection/treatment/trauma
- Previous episodes
- Previous antimicrobial treatment

Systems

- Airway – SOB, drooling
- Dental – changes in occlusion, loose teeth, difficulty chewing
- Eye – changes in vision, painful/restricted eye movements
- Face – spreading swelling/erythema, numbness/paraesthesia (especially labio-mental)
- Neurological – nausea, vomiting, headache, loss of consciousness, syncope, seizures
- Systemic – fevers, malaise

Risk factors/Red flags

- Previous dental treatment/infection
- Trauma
- Bony pathology – Paget's disease of the bone, osteopetrosis, osteogenesis imperfecta
- Immunocompromise – malignancy, diabetes, malnutrition, anaemia, HIV, corticosteroids/chemotherapy
- Smoking
- Radiation exposure

AMPLE

- Allergies, regular/recent medications, other relevant past medical history, time of last meal

Examination

- General inspection – dehydrated, cachectic, facial swelling/asymmetry, drooling
- Dentition – malocclusion, carous/broken teeth (tender to percussion)
- Face – swelling, erythema, paraesthesia, numbness (labiomental numbness)
- Oral – halitosis, trismus, fistula, swelling (floor of mouth, mucosa, tongue)
- Bone – mandibular lower border steps, mobile segments, exposed bone, expansion (tender/non-tender)
- Neck – lymphadenopathy, range of motion
- Full set of observations – assess for signs of sepsis (tachycardia, fever, hypotension)

Management

The principle of management in patients with osteomyelitis is prompt diagnosis, early treatment and exclusion of any benign or neoplastic differentials. The diagnosis is usually established through a combination of clinical, radiological and tissue examination with treatment involving a combination of non-surgical and surgical interventions. The aim of surgical treatment is to remove non-viable bone and cut back to healthy bleeding bone. Reconstruction may be required including fixation of any secondary fractures. If no fractures are present, the risk of perioperative fractures should be assessed and a decision made regarding whether fixation is required (external or plating) to prevent pathological fracture based on the extent of debridement required.

Bedside

- Swabs – mc&s
- Bloods – FBC, U&E, CRP, lactate, blood cultures, HbA1c

Imaging

- OPG – early changes may not be detectable
- CT facial bones/neck – assess extent of disease and relation to vital anatomical structures (inferior dental canal, maxillary sinus), operative planning (Figure 2.1)
- MRI – early stages of osteomyelitis as shows bone marrow changes
- Nuclear imaging (PET/SPECT) – considered in complex or refractory cases for mapping chronic infection sites

Typical radiographic findings

1) Suppurative osteomyelitis – localised radiolucent areas with ragged borders ("moth eaten"). Later stages can demonstrate radio-opaque sequestrum surrounded by radiolucent involucrum.
2) Sclerosing osteomyelitis – diffuse radiopacity (sclerosis) affecting the whole bone with loss of demarcation of lower border of the mandible and inferior dental canal. Can be associated with bony expansion due to periosteal bony reaction.
3) Garre osteomyelitis – periosteal bone formation and layered cortical expansion (onion skin appearance). Presence of the deciduous or permanent offending tooth.

Biopsy

- Tissue (medullary space)/bony sampling can lead to a definitive diagnosis – histology and microbiology

Non-surgical

- IV antibiotics – involve microbiologist
- Hyperbaric oxygen – not well established; consider as an adjunct for non-responsive chronic cases
- Managing risk factors – smoking, diabetes, immunosuppression that may affect healing

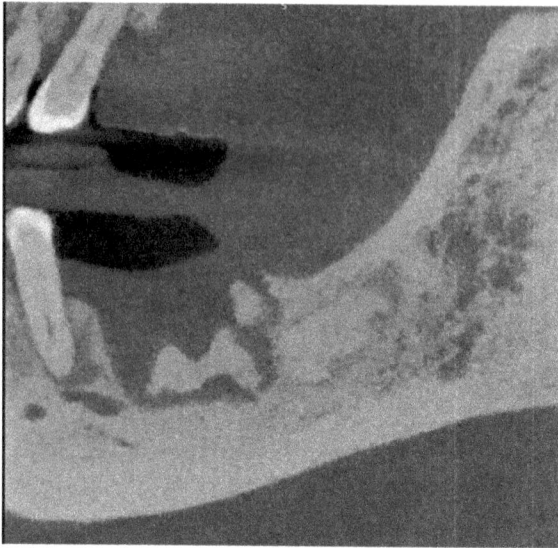

Figure 2.1 Sagittal view of cone beam CT showing chronic osteomyelitis of the body of the mandible. There is a sequestrum formation with evidence of chronic infection and granulation/ soft tissue.

- Local antibiotics (e.g., antibiotic-loaded resorbable beads) following surgical debridement

Surgical

- Keep the patient NBM
- Consent the patient by explaining the benefits, risks and alternative
- Offer surgical exploration and debridement (sequestrectomy and saucerization) of the affected area ± dental extractions
- If primary closure cannot be achieved, it is possible to pack the wound to heal by secondary intention
- May require a re-look / second-stage debridement
- Decortication – well-established treatment for chronic osteomyelitis (removal of cortical bone and the medullary bone put in direct contact with the periosteum)
- Garre osteomyelitis
  - Eradication of the cause of infection – usually posterior mandibular tooth
  - Empirical course of antibiotics
  - Usually self-limiting within 3–4 months
  - If fails to respond then perform a bone biopsy (histology) and culture and sensitivity should be considered
- In progressive cases refractive to antimicrobial treatment – consider repeat surgical debridement
- Pathological fractures or persistent labio-mental numbness are more likely to require more extensive surgical treatment (resection with immediate or delayed reconstruction)
- Consider reconstructive options in an MDT approach

Red flags

- Radiotherapy to the head and neck – risk of osteoradionecrosis
- Previous antiresorptive medication – risk of medication related osteonecrosis of the jaw
- Labiomental numbness
- Oral antral communication
- Changes in occlusion
- Weight loss
- Immunocompromise
- Malignancy with bony metastases
- Bone disorders – Paget's disease of the bone, osteoporosis, osteogenesis imperfecta
- Antiresorptive drugs – bisphosphonates or denosumab may contribute to MRONJ

MCQs

1) What is the most common cause of mandibular osteomyelitis?

   A) Haematogenous spread from a systemic infection
   B) Direct spread from a dentoalveolar infection
   C) Trauma without associated infection
   D) Prior radiation exposure to the mandible
   E) Use of antiresorptive medications such as bisphosphonates

2) Which of the following is a hallmark radiographic finding of Garre osteomyelitis?

   A) Diffuse radiopacity with periosteal bone reaction
   B) Localised radiolucent areas with ragged borders
   C) Onion-skin periosteal bone formation with layered cortical expansion
   D) Radio-opaque sequestrum surrounded by radiolucent involucrum
   E) Moth-eaten appearance of the affected bone

3) What is the first-line surgical approach for managing chronic suppurative osteomyelitis?

   A) Hyperbaric oxygen therapy
   B) Resection with immediate reconstruction
   C) Sequestrectomy and saucerization
   D) Bone biopsy and delayed reconstruction
   E) Decortication with external fixation

Chapter 3

Ludwig's angina, necrotising fasciitis and airway compromise

Salman Tahir and Peter Stockton

Background

The most significant of all head and neck infections are Ludwig's angina and necrotising fasciitis. Ludwig's angina is an extensive cellulitis involving submental, bilateral submandibular, and sublingual spaces. Necrotising fasciitis is an aggressive infection of the skin that can progress to necrosis of the muscle fascia and subcutaneous tissues due to poor blood supply of the fascial plane. While this commonly affects the abdomen, groin, perineum, and extremities, head and neck involvement can be in up to 10% of cases, with an odontogenic cause accounting for up to half of these. Complications of head and neck necrotising fasciitis may include airway compromise, arterial and venous occlusion, and mediastinal extension, as well as systemic involvement leading to organ failure, sepsis, and shock. Both conditions are surgical emergencies due to their rapid nature and, if not dealt with in a timely manner, can result in significant morbidity and mortality as a consequence of sepsis or airway compromise. Should this be the case, and patients present with life-threatening airway risk, this should be secured immediately and takes precedence over any history or examination.

Potential areas of deterioration

A risk of airway obstruction progressing to respiratory arrest and death
C septic shock

Preparation and equipment

- These are critical OMFS emergencies, and patients should be assessed immediately
- Ensure the patient is in an appropriate high-dependency area with the difficult airway equipment available
- Call the anaesthetic team and ENT to attend alongside you
- Make senior colleague aware that you have a potential airway concern

Immediate assessment

- Rapid A to E assessment before proceeding
- If the patient presents in cardiorespiratory arrest, commence CPR and resuscitation according to ALS guidelines

DOI: 10.1201/9781003493310-4

Table 3.1 Classifications of Necrotising Fasciitis

Type 1	Type 2	Type 3	Type 4
Most common	Less common	Uncommon	Rare
Polymicrobial	Monomicrobial	Monomicrobial	Fungal
Anaerobes and aerobic	Usually facultative anaerobe	Gram negative	Fungal
Bacteroides, Clostridium, Enterobacteriaceae, non-group A *Streptococcus*	*Streptococcus pyogenes, Staphylococcus aureus*	*Vibrio* spp.	Candida
Diabetics	Healthy patients following trauma/ skin breach	Seafood, water, contaminated wounds	Trauma, immunocompromise

History

Symptoms – usually mouth/neck swelling (Ludwig's angina) or skin rash (necrotising fasciitis)

- Onset, timing, and duration
- Overlying skin changes
- Better or worse
- Intermittent/continuous
- Preceding factors, e.g., dental infection/treatment/trauma
- Previous episodes (especially requiring admission to hospital/ICU)
- Known history of head and neck malignancy

Systems

- Airway – SOB, aspiration/choking, drooling
- Oesophagus – rapid onset dysphagia, odynophagia, regurgitation
- Voice – rapid onset change in voice

Risk factors/Red flags

- Recent dental infection/treatment
- Smoking, alcohol
- Diabetes, immunocompromise, liver cirrhosis, anaemia

AMPLE

- Allergies, regular/recent medications, other relevant past medical history, time of last meal

Examination

- General inspection for signs of respiratory distress – noisy breathing (stridor, stertor), tachypnoea, cyanosis, use of accessory muscles, anxiety, agitation, fatigue, drooling

- Skin – initially red developing to blue/black and progressing
- Voice – speaking in full sentences, quality of voice, hoarseness
- Neck – range of motion and torticollis, lumps, cellulitis, large diffuse bilateral neck swelling
- Oral cavity/Oropharynx – tongue and floor of mouth swelling (raised tongue), tonsils, peritonsillar swelling, halitosis, trismus
- Dentition – broken/carous teeth (tender to percussion)
- Chest – palpation for surgical emphysema and auscultation for signs of aspiration
- Full set of observations – assess for signs of respiratory distress (tachypnoea, reduced saturations) or sepsis (tachycardia, fever, hypotension)

Management

The principle of management in patients with Ludwig's angina or necrotising fasciitis is to treat the underlying infection and manage or prevent any acute airway obstruction. Ensuring a stable airway may require securing a definitive airway (endotracheal intubation or front-of-neck access) or medical management strategies that can be employed in less critical presentations.

Bedside

- Sit patient up
- Monitor saturations and oxygenate (15 L high-flow oxygen or HFNC therapy)
- Heliox can buy time if immediately available (21% oxygen, 79% helium) – has a lower density than air which improves oxygen delivery to the airways
- IV broad-spectrum antibiotics and corticosteroid if concerns about airway
- Nebulisers – adrenaline and/or corticosteroids
- Bloods – FBC, U&E, CRP, lactate, blood cultures, HbA1c

Imaging

- OPG – dental cause
- CT neck with contrast – extent of swelling, collection, gas, diffuse thickening of the subcutaneous tissue and cervical fascia (Figure 3.1), fluid collections, and airway assessment
  - Gas within fluid collections is the hallmark of necrotising fasciitis

Conservative/Medical – less likely employed

- Admit the patient for close observations
- Continue with IV antibiotics, corticosteroid, nebulisers, oxygen, heliox as indicated
- Discuss options for further management and next steps with the patient when they are stable
- Make critical care teams aware if not being admitted to ICU/HDU and have a plan for steps to be taken if the patient deteriorates

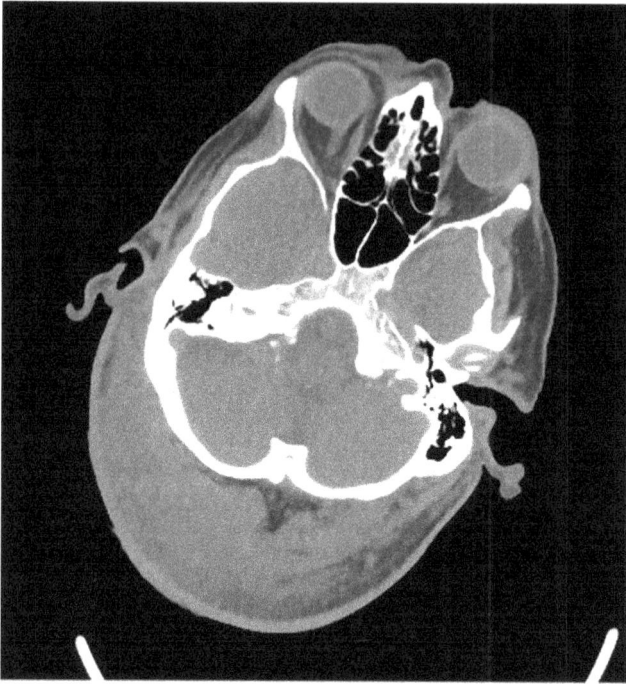

Figure 3.1 Axial CT scan showing soft tissue thickening and presence of gas in the posterior neck and occipital tissues.

Surgical and airway control

- Keep the patient NBM
- If able, consent the patient by explaining benefits, risks, and alternatives
- Work closely with the anaesthetist and have a clear plan prior to the procedure in cases of a difficult airway this could be
  - This could be facemask ventilation and endotracheal intubation (using direct laryngoscopy, video laryngoscopy, bougie or fibreoptic nasal intubation [maximum 3+1 attempts])
- Emergency front-of-neck access (FONA) should only be performed in "can't intubate, can't ventilate" scenario that may require ENT support
  - Surgical tracheostomy – preferred, safer, longer procedure
  - Scalpel cricothyroidotomy
- Transfer the patient to ICU for postoperative care and close monitoring (usually 24–48 hours)
- The decision to extubate/decannulate should be made with an MDT approach
  - Irreversible/progressive cause of airway obstruction may require a long-term tracheostomy

Ludwig's angina

- Extraoral incision and drainage / decompression of abscess / cellulitis with multiple drains
  - Swabs and cultures
- Dental extractions (source of infection)

Necrotising fasciitis

- Early and aggressive debridement of all necrotic tissue
- Be wary of normal-looking tissue that likely has early or extensive thrombosis / vasculitis
- Multiple surgeries and re-looks often required
- Dental extractions (source of infection)
- Second-stage skin reconstructions (flaps, grafts)

Discharge and follow-up

- Evidence of clinical improvement – airway, swelling, infection markers, oral intake
- Discharge with oral antibiotics and review in clinic to ensure complete recovery

MCQs

1) A 35-year-old taxi driver presents in ED with bilateral neck swelling which extends into bilateral submandibular, sublingual, and submental spaces. He is vitally stable, but sitting upright, drooling, and has a hoarseness in his voice when he tries to speak. Which of the following will be your cornerstone for initial management?

   A) Arrange for an urgent CT neck to assess for collection
   B) Inform anaesthetist on call and start taking steps to manage airway
   C) Transfer to theatre for emergency tracheostomy
   D) Transfer to theatre for incision and drainage
   E) Start immediately on IV antibiotics

2) You are called in ICU at 2 AM to review a 42-year-old patient who underwent tracheostomy for airway management followed by incision and drainage of bilateral submandibular and sublingual spaces 3 days ago. He has bilateral corrugated drains in place in the submandibular region and is currently in ICU. On examination you notice that his bilateral submandibular swelling has increased in size, and his WCC and CRP are increasing. What will be your next steps in management?

   A) Arrange for an urgent CT neck to assess for re-collection
   B) Change the tracheostomy tube
   C) Transfer to theatre for emergency re-drainage of abscess
   D) Continue with same IV antibiotics
   E) No intervention required since the patient is vitally stable

3) A middle-aged female presents to ED with left lateral submandibular neck swelling. She is poorly controlled Type 2 diabetic and is hypertensive. You have taken a detailed history and were told that swelling started 2 days ago after she got her left mandibular molar tooth extracted because of dental abscess. On examination, she has left lateral neck swelling with overlying skin which is dark blue/blackish in colour and on palpation you can feel the crepitus. Her HR is 110, BP is 105/70 mmHg, RR 20/min, temperature 37.8°C, and SpO_2 99% on room air. What will be your primary goal of management?

A) Airway management
B) IV antibiotics and fluids
C) Surgical drainage and debridement of necrotic tissue
D) Debridement of necrotic tissue and skin grafting at the same time
E) Discharge on oral antibiotic

Chapter 4

Osteonecrosis of the jaw

Sherif Amer and Shofiq Islam

Background

Osteonecrosis of the jaw has many different subtypes all of which encompass bony damage and disruption with subsequent exposed gum. It is often characterised by pain and swelling in the gums with secondary infections, loosening of teeth and oral ulcers. There can also be an associated numbness in the affected area. The main two causes of jaw osteonecrosis are medication-related osteonecrosis of the jaw (MRONJ) and osteoradionecrosis (ORN) of the jaw.

MRONJ was first described in the early 2000s and is characterised by exposed or palpable bone in the maxillofacial region persisting for over 8 weeks. By definition, it occurs in patients with a current or previous history of antiangiogenic or antiresorptive medications, and no prior history of jaw radiotherapy or metastatic disease to the jaw. MRONJ is often linked to invasive dental procedures, although trauma from dentures and spontaneous MRONJ cases have also been recognised. ORN of the jaw is a late complication of radiotherapy with exposed necrotic bone in the jaw that does not heal within 3 months with no evidence of tumour recurrence or metastasis. ORN most commonly affects the mandible and occurs due to the "three H's" of radiation-induced tissue injury: hypocellularity, hypovascularity and hypoxia.

History

Symptoms – can be variable (pain, swelling, infection)

- Onset, timing and duration
- Laterality
- Progression
- Ability to maintain adequate oral intake
- Preceding events – radiotherapy, malignancy, antiresorptive medication, trauma, infection, dental work
- Previous episodes

Systems

- Dental – changes in occlusion, loose teeth, difficulty chewing, halitosis, dental infections, loose teeth
- Face – spreading swelling/erythema, numbness/paraesthesia
- Systemic – fevers

DOI: 10.1201/9781003493310-5

Past medical history

- Head and neck cancer and treatment (specifically radiotherapy including date of last cycle and dose)
- Diabetes
- Immunocompromise

Drug history – important in MRONJ (Table 4.1)

- Specifically ask about known medications that can cause MRONJ including dose, route and length of treatment
  - Antiresorptive (bisphosphonates, RANKL inhibitors, sclerostin inhibitors)
  - Antiangiogenic (bevacizumab, sunitinib, aflibercept)
  - Immune checkpoint inhibitors (pembrolizumab)
  - Protein kinase inhibitors
  - Combination therapy

Social history

- Smoking, alcohol status
- Performance status
- Impact on quality of life, activities of daily living and hobbies including social/ public eating

Risk factors

MRONJ

- Low risk
  - Oral or IV bisphosphonates or denosumab for osteoporosis or benign conditions for <5 years without concurrent steroid therapy
  - Off denosumab for more than 9 months

- High risk
  - Antiresorptive medications for >5 years
  - Antiresorptive-steroid combinations
  - Combined antiresorptive and antiangiogenic drugs
  - Prior MRONJ history
  - Oncology patients

ORN

- Higher risk
  - First 3 years post-radiotherapy
  - Direct irradiation of mandible (rare in maxilla)
  - Radiotherapy doses above 60 Gy
  - Large tumours (e.g., T4)
  - Dental extractions
  - Oropharyngeal and oral cavity cancers

- Lower risk
  - IMRT (intensity-modulated radiation therapy) and proton and particle therapies may minimise risk through reduced doses

Table 4.1 Common Medications Implicated in MRONJ

Class	Common Drugs	Mechanism	Half-Life and Persistence	Risk of MRONJ (Osteoporosis)	Risk of MRONJ (Cancer)
Bisphosphonates	Alendronate, Zoledronate, Ibandronate	Bind to bone hydroxyapatite, inhibiting osteoclast activity and reducing bone turnover; some antiangiogenic effects affecting soft tissue healing	Binds to bone; alendronate half-life ~10 years	0.02%–0.05%	1–5%
RANKL Inhibitors	Denosumab	Inhibits RANK ligand, reducing osteoclast formation and function	No bone binding; effects diminish within 9 months post-therapy	0.04%–0.3%	N/A
Sclerostin Inhibitors	Romosozumab	Inhibits sclerostin, increasing bone formation and reducing resorption	Effect weakens after 12 months	0.03%–0.05%	N/A

Examination

- Facial asymmetry/Disfigurement
- Halitosis
- Mandibular fractures
- Full systematic examination of the oral cavity (Figure 4.1)
  - Exposed bone – not healing after 8 weeks of appropriate treatment is sensitive for osteonecrosis of the jaw
  - Swelling and tenderness
  - Loose teeth – secondary to bone destruction
  - Purulent drainage – from gums around exposed bone
  - Fistula – oro-nasal, oro-antral, extraoral
  - Lip/facial paraesthesia/numbness

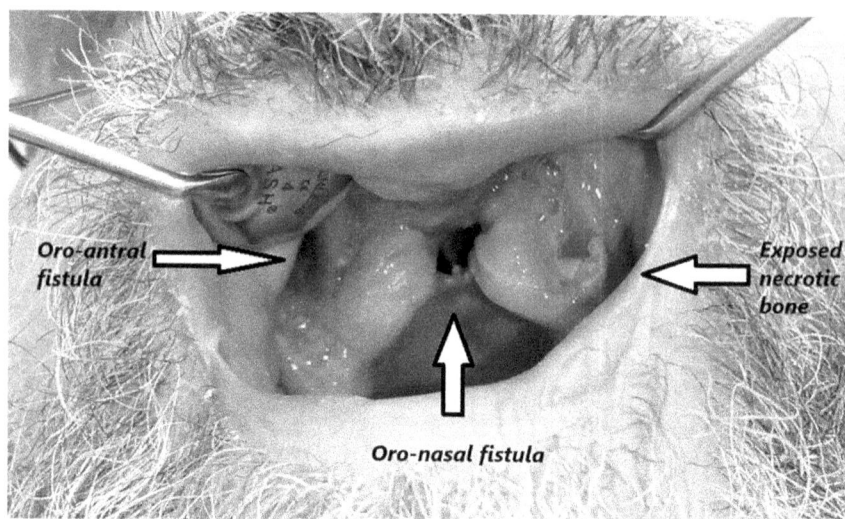

Figure 4.1 Maxillary MRONJ in a multiple myeloma patient on zoledronate, presenting with pain, exposed bone in the left maxilla, bone necrosis leading to large midline oro-nasal fistula and an oro-antral fistula in the right buccal sulcus. Temporary prosthesis fabrication was required to facilitate oral intake and effective phonation.

Management

The principles of management in patients with jaw osteonecrosis is to control risk factors, educate patients, minimise further risk and complication and support patient quality of life through pain management, infection control and preventing disease progression. The balance of avoiding osteonecrosis progression while maintaining treatment in malignancy can be difficult and requires close follow-up and an MDT approach with OMFS, oral surgeons/dentists, oncologists and hygienists. Additionally, osteonecrosis significantly impacts quality of life by impairing nutrition, speech and emotional well-being. A multidisciplinary approach, incorporating psychological support and patient-centred care, is essential in managing this physical and psychological burden. For MRONJ, priority should be given to minimising MRONJ risk to avoid treatment interruption for osteoporosis or cancer therapy. Patients should be informed that the overall MRONJ risk is low, and that generally, the benefits of treatment outweigh the risks. Before initiating antiresorptive therapy, all high-risk procedures (e.g., extractions of teeth with poor prognosis) should be completed to prevent MRONJ. If systemic conditions permit, antiresorptive initiation should be delayed until dental health is stabilised.

General preventative measures

- Control periodontal disease and caries
- Dietary advice to maintain optimal oral hygiene
- Fluoride prescriptions as needed
- Encourage smoking cessation, alcohol reduction
- Control modifiable risk factors – e.g., diabetes
- Avoid trauma
- Ensure proper fitting of dentures and other prostheses to minimise mucosal trauma
- Discontinuing antiresorptive drugs before dentoalveolar surgery is no longer recommended
- Low- and high-risk patients may undergo unavoidable extractions in primary care settings, followed by monitoring

MRONJ

- When possible, prioritise ongoing cancer or osteoporosis treatment, though a temporary drug suspension may be considered based on patient needs and with prescriber input
- Stage-based approach to treatment in MRONJ (Table 4.2)
- Adjunct therapies
  - Vitamin E and pentoxifylline
  - Teriparatide
  - Hyperbaric oxygen and ozone therapy (use is experimental/contentious)

ORN

- During radiotherapy
  - Protective shields can minimise risk of ORN
  - Symptomatic management – pain control, antibiotics, avoid dental extractions if possible
  - Jaw exercises – reduce radiation-related trismus risk

- After radiotherapy
  - Complete necessary extractions within 4 months post-radiotherapy (before chronic ORN-inducing hypoxia, hypovascularity and hypocellularity)
  - Unavoidable extractions should be performed by specialists, especially for patients who received >60 Gy
  - Antibiotic prophylaxis is advised for extractions or sequestrectomy to prevent infection until full mucosal coverage is achieved
  - Regularly inspect dentures and prostheses, as mucosal trauma may precipitate ORN

Table 4.2 Stage-Based Approach to MRONJ Management

Stage	Presentation	Management
At Risk	No necrotic bone; asymptomatic patients with IV or oral antiresorptive or antiangiogenic therapy	Patient education Regular dental checkups (every 3–6 months) Avoid dentoalveolar surgery if possible
Stage 0	No exposed bone, but possible unexplained pain, tooth mobility, or dull ache; radiographic changes (e.g., sclerosis)	Antibacterial mouth rinse Close clinical follow-up Patient education and management of modifiable risk factors
Stage I	Exposed or necrotic bone, asymptomatic without infection, localised radiographic changes	Analgesics Antibacterial mouth rinse Close follow-up with OMFS specialist
Stage II	Exposed necrotic bone with infection/purulence or pain	Analgesics Antibacterial mouth rinse Oral antibiotics Surgical debridement may be considered for persistent symptoms
Stage III	Necrotic bone with advanced infection, with fracture, fistulas or sinus involvement	Operative management (surgical debridement/resective surgery with reconstruction with local flap or free tissue transfer)

- **Non-surgical management**
  - Antibiotics – systemic or topical
  - Analgesia
  - Nutritional support
  - PENTO/PENTOCLO protocols – consider pentoxifylline (800 mg) and vitamin E (1,000 IU), with or without clodronate, for up to 6 months or longer if improvement is observed
  - Low-level laser therapy (LLLT) – pain reduction, healing promotion, trismus relief
  - Radioprotective agents – amifostine has shown early potential in reducing radiation injury to bone

- **Surgical management**
  - Sequestrectomy or saucerisation – local removal of necrotic bone can aid healing and prevent further deterioration
  - Advanced interventions – in severe cases partial or complete resection of the mandible or maxilla may be required, with reconstruction using free flaps to restore both form and function (Figures 4.2–4.4)

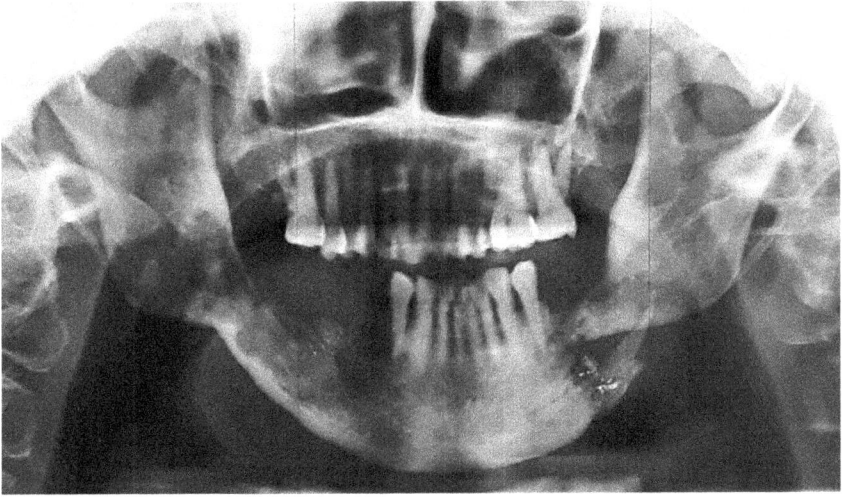

Figure 4.2 Panoramic radiograph (OPG) showing bilateral Notani Stage III ORN with mandibular fractures post-radiotherapy for an advanced tongue base malignancy.

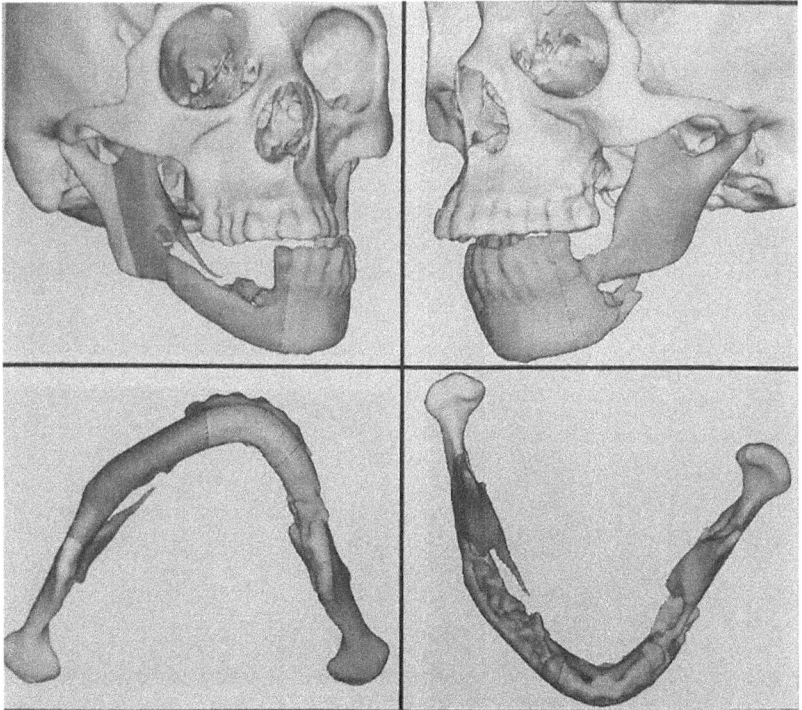

Figure 4.3 Bilateral ORN-associated mandibular fractures with malocclusion and facial deformity. Pre-surgical planning utilising CAD/CAM for bilateral segmental resection and reconstruction using a double-paddled osteo cutaneous free fibular flap.

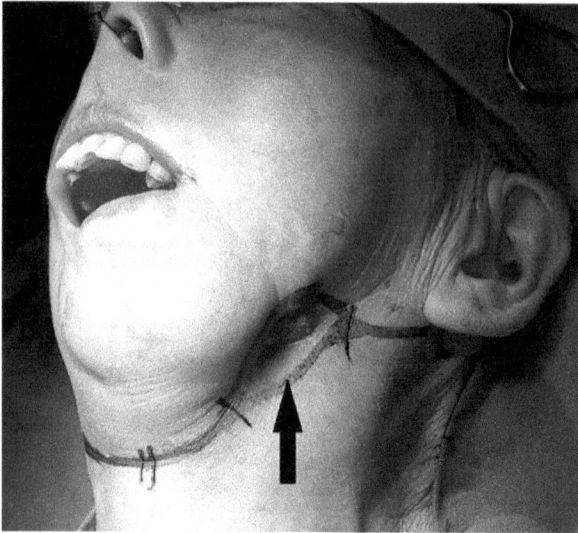

Figure 4.4 Intraoperative image of patient with bilateral pathological fractures of mandible (Stage III ORN), overt facial disfigurement and a large extraoral fistula (black arrow).

Lyons system classifying of established osteoradionecrosis

- *Stage 1*: Bone involvement <2.5 cm, asymptomatic, managed medically
- *Stage 2*: Bone involvement >2.5 cm with asymptomatic complications, such as pathologic fracture, managed medically unless infection is present
- *Stage 3*: >2.5 cm bone involvement with symptoms, consider surgical debridement
- *Stage 4*: Advanced involvement with complications requiring reconstruction if the patient's condition permits

MCQs

1) Which of the following is NOT a risk factor for MRONJ?

    A) Long-term use of bisphosphonates for osteoporosis
    B) Combined use of antiresorptive and antiangiogenic drugs
    C) Radiation therapy to the jaw
    D) Trauma from poorly fitting dentures
    E) Recent dental extractions

2) Which stage of MRONJ is characterised by exposed or necrotic bone with infection or purulence and associated pain?

    A) At risk
    B) Stage 0
    C) Stage I
    D) Stage II
    E) Stage III

3) What is the primary mechanism by which bisphosphonates contribute to the development of MRONJ?

    A) Inhibition of osteoclast activity and reduced bone turnover
    B) Increased vascularity in bone tissue
    C) Stimulation of osteoblast function
    D) Direct suppression of immune response
    E) Enhanced soft tissue healing

Mandibular trauma

Zahra Al Asaadi and Prav Praveen

Background

Fractures of the mandible can occur in isolation or in the context of polytrauma and head injuries. Since the advent of legislation regarding seat belt use, the incidence of mandibular trauma due to road traffic accidents has reduced and a fracture of the mandible is most commonly due to interpersonal trauma, sporting incidents and, increasingly, falls especially in an ageing population. The mandible is a U-shaped bone with the condylar head on each side part of the temporo-mandibular joint. Fractures of the mandible are divided according to the region involved – the symphysis and parasymphysis, the body, the angle and the condyle. Due to its unique anatomy multiple fractures of the mandible are common. The most frequent fracture pattern involves a fracture of the parasymphysis with a contralateral angle or condylar fracture. If the fracture involves the tooth-bearing portion of the mandible, this is classified as an open fracture due to communication of the fracture site with the oral cavity and would require antibiotic cover. There may be associated dental injury or teeth involved in the fracture line that may be loose or fractured and should be accounted for.

Potential areas of deterioration

A   loose or fractured teeth may be an airway risk especially in a polytrauma patient who may have intracranial injuries and is unable to protect their airway

Preparation and equipment

- OMFS may be asked to attend as part of the formal trauma team in the event of polytrauma; a full OMFS assessment is important in an ATLS approach
  - The team should attend early to introduce themselves, assign roles and receive handover from the pre-hospital team if the patient is brought in by ambulance
  - Ensure the patient is assessed in accordance with ATLS protocol with a primary survey
  - Deal with any other potential injuries in order of priority according to trauma scenario
- If this is an isolated injury, the patient should be assessed for any head injury prior to acceptance by the OMFS team

DOI: 10.1201/9781003493310-6

- They should be assessed the same day either in ED or on a ward if the fracture is displaced

History

Event

- Preceding events
- Localisation of pain and swelling
- Type of event leading to the trauma – assault, sporting injury, fall
- Post-event – loss of consciousness, vomiting, amnesia

Systems

- Airway – SOB, aspiration/choking, drooling
- Dental – malocclusion
- Facial – paraesthesia/numbness
- Neurological – loss of consciousness or other neurological symptoms

Risk factors/Red flags

- History of malignancy or suspicion of pathological fracture
- Features of high impact trauma and risk of head injury
- Inability to account for missing teeth

AMPLE

- Allergies, regular medications, other relevant medical history, time of last meal
- Drugs/alcohol consumption

Examination

- General inspection – active bleeding, consciousness level
- Respiratory distress – noisy breathing (stridor, stertor), tachypnoea, cyanosis, use of accessory muscles, anxiety, agitation, fatigue
- Full assessment of facial bones
- Jaw – TMJ tenderness, mouth opening, trismus, extraoral lacerations
- Oral cavity – occlusion, step deformities, sublingual haematoma (may be a sign of fracture), missing or fractured teeth
- Cranial nerves – especially V and VII
- Full set of observations

Management

The principle of managing a fractured mandible is to aim for bony healing and restoration of the occlusion of the patient. Undisplaced fractures may be initially managed conservatively with a soft diet but require early review to ensure they have not become displaced. The principles of managing a displaced fracture include reduction of the fracture and fixation. This can be done either with an open approach with titanium miniplates using the principles of osteosynthesis or a closed approach using intermaxillary fixation (wiring of the jaws). The advent

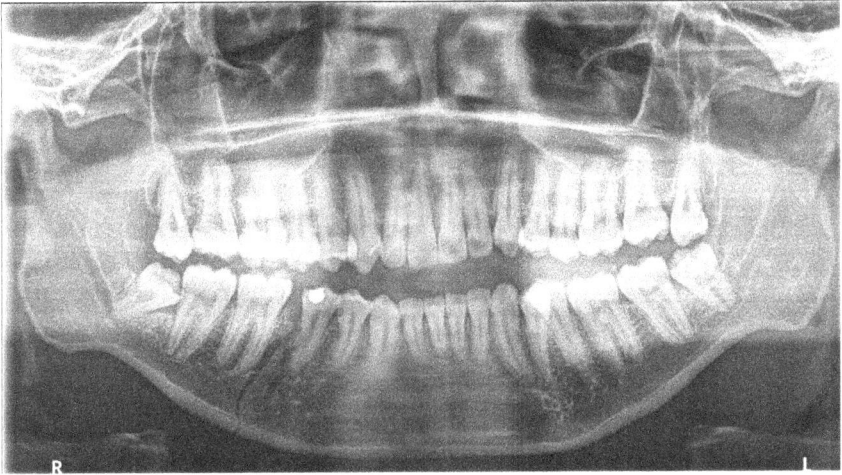

Figure 5.1 OPG showing mandibular fracture of the right parasymphysis and left condyle.

of titanium miniplates has allowed for rapid fracture healing using small plates to reduce facial fractures.

Bedside investigations

- Routine blood tests are rarely indicated
- FBC, U&Es, coagulation profile, group an save/crossmatch can be taken part of the surgical workup

Imaging

- Plain radiographs require two views – OPG/DPT (Figure 5.1) and a PA mandible view
- CT mandible – indicated for complex or comminuted fractures, mandibular condyle fractures or assessing multiple facial fractures

Medical

- Prophylactic IV antibiotics until fixation if an open and displaced fracture
- Analgesia

Surgical (Figure 5.2)

- Keep the patient NBM
- Informed consent of the patient discussing risks, benefits and alternatives
- Surgical intervention for displaced fractures when next available on the emergency list
- Open reduction and internal fixation of the fracture(s) ± use of intermaxillary fixation (IMF) with adjuncts such as archbars to the teeth or IMF screws with postoperative elastics to guide the patient's occlusion
- Displaced condylar fractures need a separate extraoral incision

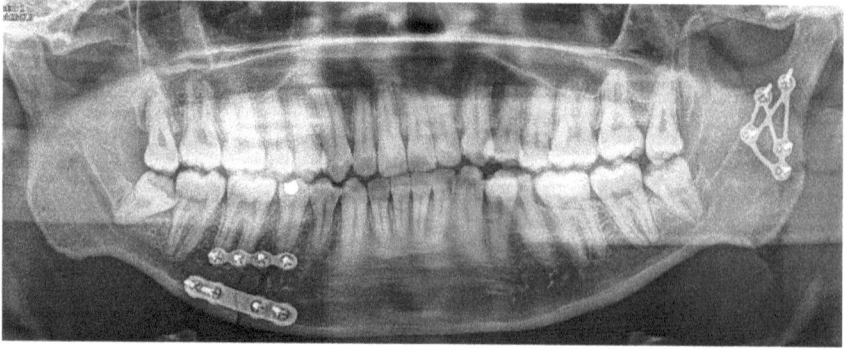

Figure 5.2 OPG following ORIF for bilateral mandibular fractures.

Discharge and follow-up

- Undisplaced fracture – advise to have a soft/liquid diet for 4–6 weeks with close weekly follow-up
- Postoperatively – once occlusion confirmed and radiographs confirm reduction, soft/liquid diet 4–6 weeks
- Some patients may require postoperative elastics for a few weeks to guide their teeth into the correct position
- Initial follow-up should be weekly, with discharge following confirmation of healing and no infection (usually 6 weeks postoperatively)

Red flags/Complicated fractures

- Pathological fractures of the mandible
  - Malignancy
  - Osteoradionecrosis of the mandible secondary to radiotherapy or medication
- Edentulous patients – often require extraoral fixation
- Postoperative healing can be affected by
  - Immunocompromise
  - Smoking
  - Poor compliance with postoperative instructions
  - Poor oral hygiene
- Poor healing can result in non- or mal-union or plate infection

MCQs

1) Which nerve may be affected by a fracture through the angle of the mandible?

   A) Marginal mandibular nerve
   B) Infraorbital nerve
   C) Inferior alveolar nerve
   D) Buccal branch of the facial nerve
   E) Zygomatic nerve

2) Which of the following statements about fractured mandibles is FALSE?

   A) Undisplaced fractures of the condyle can be managed conservatively
   B) A displaced fracture through the mandibular parasymphysis does not require antibiotics
   C) An open reduction of the mandibular condyle may cause facial weakness
   D) Teeth involved in a fracture may require extraction
   E) There is a risk to the vagus nerve during ORIF

3) Which statement about assessment for a fractured mandible is FALSE?

   A) Maxillofacial trauma should be assessed according to ATLS principles
   B) High-impact trauma should raise suspicion for other injuries
   C) Sublingual haematoma is a sign that a fracture of the mandible is present
   D) Mandibles often fracture in more than one location
   E) Road traffic accidents are the most common cause of a fractured mandible

Chapter 6

Midface trauma

Zahra Al Asaadi and Prav Praveen

Background

The midface consists of the maxilla, the bones that make up the zygomatic complex and the orbit. Trauma to the midface most commonly occurs due to interpersonal trauma, road traffic accidents, sporting injuries and falls. The injuries may occur in isolation or as part of pan-facial fractures or alongside intracranial, base-of-skull and cervical spine injuries. There are areas of strength that provide bony support for the midface – the anterior (nasomaxillary) buttresses and the zygomaticomaxillary buttresses – and areas of weakness including the maxillary sinuses. The maxilla contains the tooth-bearing portion of the midface.

The zygomatic complex may be fractured in one or multiple locations including at the frontozygomatic suture, the zygomatic arch and the orbital rim. The orbital floor itself may fracture in isolation without involving the orbital rim in a 'trap-door' fashion with the orbital contents herniating through the floor into the maxillary antrum. Entrapment of muscle (usually inferior rectus) or orbital fat can result in diplopia and restriction of upward gaze. Longer term, enophthalmos may result. Bilateral fractures of the midface can also occur and are often also classified according to the Le Fort classification (Table 6.1).

Potential areas of deterioration

A   teeth displacement or excess bleeding can cause potential airway compromise
C   maxillary or midface fractures may cause excess bleeding leading to hypovolaemic shock

Preparation and equipment

- OMFS may be asked to attend as part of the formal trauma team in the event of polytrauma; a full OMFS assessment is important in an ATLS approach
  - The team should attend early to introduce themselves, assign roles and receive handover from the pre-hospital team if the patient is brought in by ambulance
  - Ensure the patient is assessed in accordance with ATLS protocol with a primary survey
  - Deal with any other potential injuries in order of priority according to trauma scenario

DOI: 10.1201/9781003493310-7

Table 6.1 Summary and Description of Le Fort Fractures

	Description	Clinical	Radiology	Summary
Le Fort I	Horizontal maxillary fracture separating teeth from upper face	Malocclusion, buccal ecchymosis, epistaxis, maxilla crepitus and mobility	Fracture line passes through alveolar ridge, inferior maxillary sinus wall and lateral nose	Floating palate
Le Fort II	Pyramidal fracture with a floating maxilla	Ecchymosis (buccal, periorbital, subconjunctival), bilateral epistaxis, infraorbital paraesthesia, midface crepitus and facial lengthening	Fracture arch passes through posterior alveolar ridge, lateral maxillary sinus walls, inferior orbital rim and nasal bones (nasofrontal suture is pyramid apex)	Floating maxilla
Le Fort III	Floating transverse fracture with craniofacial disjunction	Ecchymosis (buccal, periorbital, subconjunctival), caved in or flattened face, CSF rhinorrhoea, bilateral epistaxis, lateral orbital rim defect	Transverse fracture line through nasofrontal and maxillofrontal sutures, orbital wall and zygomatic arch	Floating face

History

Event

- Preceding events
- Type of event – road traffic accident, assault
- Post-event – blood loss, loss of consciousness, seizure, amnesia

Systems

- Airway – SOB, aspiration/choking, drooling, ability to maintain airway
- Dental – malocclusion, missing teeth
- Eye – change in vision, loss of vision, double vision, bleeding
- Face – swelling, pain, asymmetry, paraesthesia/anaesthesia
- Neurological – headaches, syncope, seizures, loss of consciousness, vomiting
- Nose – nasal trauma – deviation, epistaxis, clear rhinorrhoea

Red flags/Risk factors

- High-impact trauma
- Signs of retrobulbar haemorrhage
- Signs of white eye blowout fracture

AMPLE

- Allergies, regular/recent medications, other relevant past medical history, time of last meal

Examination

- General signs of facial fracture – soft tissue bruising, swelling, bilateral periorbital bruising (racoon eyes)
- Midface or maxilla – mobility (may indicate Le Fort fractures), bony steps, discontinuity
- Eye – proptosis, visual acuity, diplopia, subconjunctival haemorrhage, ocular motility/restriction, pupil size and reaction to light, RAPD
- Oral cavity – occlusion, dental injuries, mandibular trauma
- Full set of observations

Management

The principles of management of midface injuries are to try to restore normal facial function and cosmesis. This can be achieved with conservative or surgical management. Many non-displaced zygomatic or orbital floor fractures without entrapment of orbital contents can be managed conservatively. Isolated maxillary sinus wall fractures are almost always managed conservatively with advice to avoid nose blowing because this may cause surgical emphysema.

Operative management may be indicated immediately within 24 hours, especially in cases in which there may be an airway concern or in white eye orbital floor fractures. Otherwise, in most cases, fractures are repaired 7–21 days post-injury once facial swelling and oedema have receded but prior to the onset of bony healing. The principles of management include reduction of the fracture and fixation with miniplates or in the case of an orbital floor fracture, a titanium orbital floor plate or less often a PDS sheet that supports the orbital contents once released from the defect. Any fracture involving the orbit should also have an ophthalmology assessment and will require an orthoptic assessment with a Hess chart. This measures eye movements and diplopia.

Bedside investigations

- Routine blood tests are rarely indicated
- FBC, U&Es, coagulation profile, group and save/crossmatch can be taken part of the surgical workup
- Dental impressions and study models – in Le Fort fractures to replicate original occlusion. These may be applied during surgery to allow for placement of the teeth in MMF and act as a reference point for fracture reduction

Imaging

- Plain radiographs – isolated zygomatic arch or simple zygomatic fracture
- CT facial bones – complex zygomatic fractures, orbital floor fractures, Le Fort fractures
- 3D reconstruction – helpful in planning reduction (Figure 6.1)

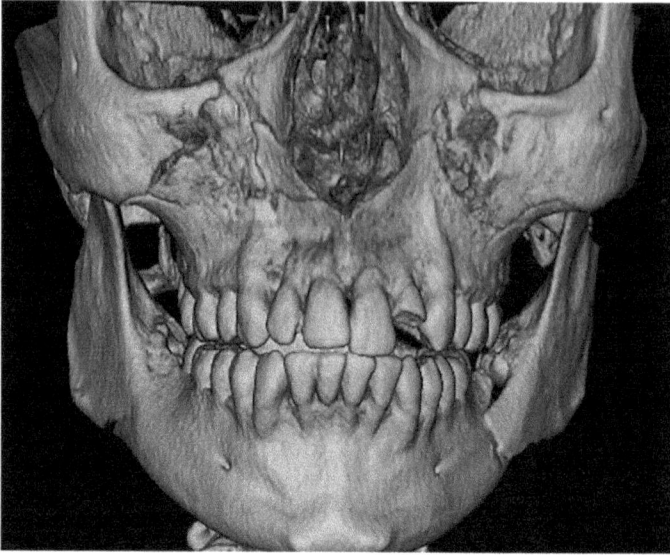

Figure 6.1 **3D CT reconstruction showing a Le Fort II fracture.**

Medical

- Consider tetanus booster or tranexamic acid if indicated
- IV antibiotics – not usually indicated in closed fractures but may be considered if overlying facial lacerations are present, especially if contaminated
- Analgesia

Surgical

- Often occurs 1–2 weeks post-injury to allow for swelling to settle but prior to bony healing
- Consider specialist anaesthetic input if submental intubation is required (if oral/nasal intubation contraindicated because the teeth need to be in occlusion)
- Incisions
  - Intraoral vestibular – access to the maxilla and zygomatic buttress
  - Scalp and lateral brow – reduce the zygoma and fracture fixation
  - Subciliary and transconjunctival – access the orbital floor
  - Bicoronal – pan-facial fractures to gain access to lateral and superior orbits and zygomatic arches
- Titanium miniplates may be placed and screwed once fracture is reduced
- Postoperative – antibiotics, steroids, regular eye observations are usually undertaken for 8 hours postoperatively in zygomatic and orbital repairs

Discharge and follow-up

- Discharge on same day with outpatient review in 1 week for further assessment and consideration of surgery – if no immediate surgery is planned (and no other injuries)
- Patients are usually discharged the next day with maxillofacial trauma clinic follow-up
- Patients should be advised not to blow their nose

Retrobulbar haemorrhage

Signs

- Severe pain
- Proptosis
- Progressive loss of vision and pupil dilatation
- Swelling of the eyelids
- Raised intraocular pressure

Complications

- Irreversible changes within optic nerve
- Loss of vision

Management

- Surgical decompression
- Lateral canthotomy and cantholysis

Paediatric white eye blowout fracture

Signs

- Excessive pain
- Vomiting
- Inability to look upward
- Diplopia (persistent)

Management

- Immediate exploration and release of entrapped muscle following orbital floor fracture

MCQs

1) Restriction of upward gaze and diplopia in orbital floor fractures often result following the entrapment of which ocular muscle?

   A) Superior oblique
   B) Inferior rectus
   C) Inferior oblique
   D) Superior rectus
   E) Levator palpebrae superioris

2) A 38-year-old male patient presents following an assault to the midface. He has significant infraorbital and cheek bruising but normal visual acuity, no diplopia and no restriction of eye movement. On examination you can palpate a step at the left infraorbital rim and he has paraesthesia of the left cheek. His teeth appear to meet as normal. What is the most likely injury?

   A) Orbital floor blowout fracture
   B) Zygomatic complex fracture
   C) Le Fort I fracture pattern
   D) Le Fort II fracture pattern
   E) Superior orbital roof fracture

3) You are asked to see a patient in recovery 2 hours after an orbital floor fracture repair. He is complaining of pain, HR is 100 and visual acuity is 6/36. On examination of the operative site the eyelids are swollen, and the globe is tense on palpation. What is the most appropriate next step?

   A) Administer analgesia
   B) Prescribe steroids
   C) Recheck eye observations in 30 minutes
   D) Prepare for a return to theatre
   E) Prescribe fluids

Chapter 7

Orbital trauma

Ahmed Abdelrahman

Background

Orbital trauma, whether isolated or associated with other facial injuries, is relatively common. Isolated orbital trauma accounts for approximately 4% to 16% of all facial injuries, while orbital fractures occur in up to 55% of cases involving facial fractures. These fractures can involve any of the four orbital walls – roof, floor, medial, or lateral walls – but are most frequently seen in the orbital floor and medial wall due to their thinner, more fragile nature. The orbit is a complex anatomical structure that houses vital structures including the eye, optic nerve, ocular muscles, and blood vessels. Given the proximity of the orbit to the brain and its connection to vital sensory and motor pathways, any trauma to this region can have severe consequences, ranging from vision loss to disfigurement, and even life-threatening complications. The eye is highly sensitive to changes in orbital volume. Trauma can lead to a reduction in this volume, causing an increase in intraorbital pressure – a situation that may lead to orbital compartment syndrome, a surgical emergency.

Complications of orbital trauma

1) **Retrobulbar haemorrhage** – sight-threatening emergency caused by bleeding behind the eye, leading to increased intraorbital pressure
2) **Orbital compartment syndrome** – ophthalmic emergency with proptosis, severe pain, and decreased vision requiring immediate surgical decompression via lateral canthotomy and inferior cantholysis to relieve pressure and prevent permanent vision loss
3) **Blindness, reduced/double vision** – resulting from damage to the optic nerve, ocular muscles, or surrounding structures
4) **Globe displacement and aesthetic concerns** – including enophthalmos, exophthalmos, and vertical dystopia
5) **Neurogenic complications** – such as nerve damage leading to sensory or motor deficits in the face and eye
6) **White eye syndrome** – a paediatric condition in which a seemingly minor orbital injury leads to severe muscle entrapment and rapid necrosis, requiring immediate intervention

DOI: 10.1201/9781003493310-8

Preparation and equipment

- OMFS may be asked to attend as part of the formal trauma team in the event of polytrauma; a full OMFS assessment is important in an ATLS approach
  - The team should attend early to introduce themselves, assign roles, and receive handover from the pre-hospital team if the patient is brought in by ambulance
  - Ensure the patient is assessed in accordance with ATLS protocol with a primary survey
  - Deal with any other potential injuries in order of priority according to trauma scenario
- If this is an isolated injury, the patient should be assessed for any head injury prior to acceptance by the OMFS team
- They should be assessed the same day either in ED due to the time-critical nature of these fractures

History

Event

- Preceding events
- Localisation of pain and swelling
- Type of event leading to the trauma – assault, sporting injury, fall
- Post-event – loss of consciousness, vomiting, amnesia

Systems

- Facial – paraesthesia/numbness
- Neurological – headaches, syncope, seizures, loss of consciousness, vomiting
- Ocular – vision changes (including colour), eye movement difficulties, pupil responses, corneal abrasion, penetrating injuries

Risk factors/Red flags

- Signs of retrobulbar haemorrhage – proptosis, reduced vision, loss of colour vision
- Signs of white eye syndrome – vomiting, bradycardia (in paediatric patients)
- Features of high-impact trauma and risk of head injury
- Inability to account for missing teeth

AMPLE

- Allergies, regular medications, other relevant medical history, time of last meal
- Drugs/alcohol consumption

Examination

- General inspection – active bleeding, consciousness level
- Facial assessment – bruising, swelling, bony steps, altered sensation
- Ophthalmological assessment – signs of trauma, visual acuity, ocular motility (mechanical entrapment vs muscle paresis), pupillary responses, globe position (enophthalmos, exophthalmos, vertical dystopia)

- Formal HESS chart assessment if diplopia suspected
- Hertel exophthalmometer can be used to document disparity between eyes
- Ophthalmology input – fundoscopy
- Cranial nerves – full examination especially II, III, IV, VI
- Neurological – if signs of intracranial injury
- Full set of observations

Management

The principle of managing orbital trauma revolves around the identification and treatment of conditions that pose an immediate threat to vision. Prompt identification and treatment of these fractures are essential, particularly in paediatric patients, in whom rapid muscle necrosis can occur within hours, leading to long-term complications if not addressed in time. Timely diagnosis and intervention are critical in preserving vision, maintaining facial aesthetics, and preventing long-term neurological or functional deficits. A multidisciplinary approach is often necessary to ensure comprehensive care and optimal outcomes including OMFS, ophthalmology, orthoptics, plastic surgery, and neurosurgery. Depending on the severity of the injury, management may occur in an inpatient or outpatient setting.

Bedside investigations

- Routine blood tests may be indicated

Imaging (Figure 7.1)

- Non-contrast CT orbit – location, size and extent of orbital fractures
- 3D CT reconstruction – surgical planning
- MRI – soft tissue components of the orbit or when CT is inconclusive – muscle or nerve involvement

Medical

- Prophylactic IV antibiotics until fixation if an open and displaced fracture
- Analgesia
- Corticosteroids – postoperative swelling

Surgical indications and timings

- Large fractures
- Significant globe displacement
- Muscle entrapment
- Typically occurs within 1–2 weeks
- Urgent cases require immediate attention

Surgical

- Keep the patient NBM
- Informed consent of the patient discussing risks, benefits, and alternatives
- Reconstruction of the orbital walls may involve the use of synthetic implants or autogenous grafts to restore normal orbital volume and prevent complications like enophthalmos

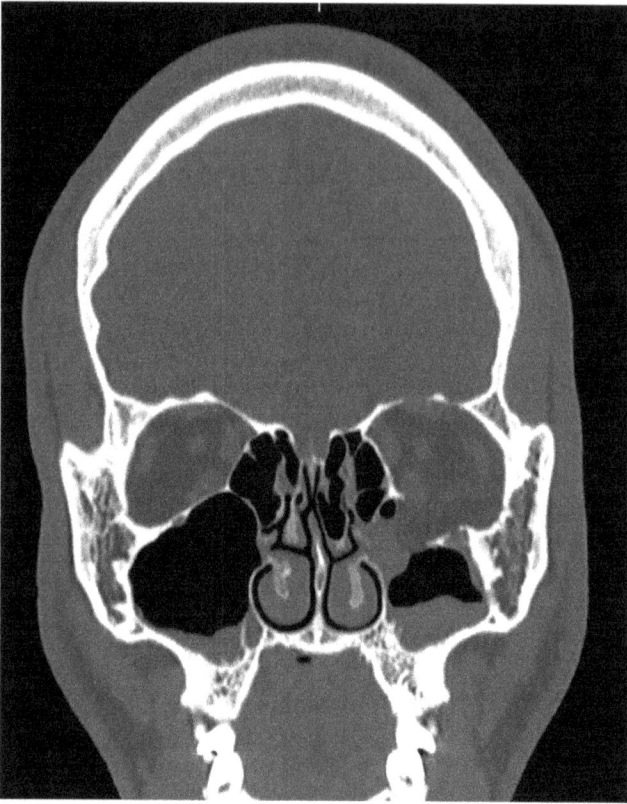

Figure 7.1 Coronal CT showing left orbital floor fracture.

Discharge and follow-up

- Discharge home once all trauma-related issues are dealt with
- Follow-up with OMFS, ophthalmology, orthoptics – regular input to monitor healing, check for complications, ensure satisfactory visual and aesthetic outcomes
- Further intervention – persistent diplopia or motility issues
- Psychosocial support – significant trauma, disfigurement, vision loss

Paediatric considerations

- Treatment urgency – paediatric patients are at higher risk for muscle necrosis following entrapment
- Follow-up – closer monitoring for potential growth-related complications, such as asymmetry or facial deformity

MCQs

1) Which of the following is considered a surgical emergency in orbital trauma?

   A) Enophthalmos with mild displacement
   B) Retrobulbar haemorrhage causing orbital compartment syndrome
   C) White eye syndrome with normal eye movement
   D) Vertical dystopia without signs of muscle entrapment
   E) Subconjunctival haemorrhage with no vision loss

2) What is the most appropriate initial imaging modality for diagnosing orbital fractures?

   A) Contrast-enhanced CT orbit
   B) MRI orbit
   C) Non-contrast CT orbit
   D) X-ray of the orbit
   E) Ultrasound

3) What is a key distinguishing feature of white eye syndrome in paediatric orbital trauma?

   A) Proptosis and severe pain
   B) Bradycardia and vomiting despite minimal external signs of injury
   C) Significant enophthalmos with vertical dystopia
   D) Severe bleeding and vision loss
   E) Paraesthesia with diplopia

Chapter 8

Frontal bone trauma
Niall M.H. McLeod

Background

Frontal bone trauma is commonly assumed to be involving the frontal sinus (Figure 8.1), since any fracture not involving this can be considered skull vault trauma and has no specific OMFS considerations unless it involves the orbit, which is managed on its own merit. Increased pneumatization of the frontal bone results in thinner bony anterior and posterior walls, but its concave shape makes it relatively strong, and relatively high-impact trauma is required for it to fracture. Such injuries are not infrequently associated with polytrauma, and in particular intracranial and cervical spine injuries. They may also be associated with other fractures of the facial skeleton. There are several classification systems for fractures of the frontal bone, but these are overly complex and fractures are best classified as involving the anterior wall, involving the posterior wall or involving the floor and frontal sinus outflow tract, or any combination thereof. Each area has its own considerations in terms of consequences, treatment options and risks.

Anterior wall fractures are predominantly cosmetic injuries, with a visible indentation in the frontal area overlying a depressed fracture. Very displaced fractures may produce obstruction to the sinus outflow. Posterior wall fractures, when significantly displaced, can be associated with dural tears and CSF rhinorrhoea and with intracranial haemorrhage. Fractures involving the outflow tract can result in mucous retention and mucocele formation. Both posterior wall and outflow tract injuries can create an increased risk of sinus disease, and ultimately intracerebral infection.

Potential areas for deterioration

D risks of intracerebral haemorrhage and infection associated with CSF fistulae or frontal sinus infection

Preparation and equipment

• This is not a true OMFS emergency because the acute problems associated with such injuries are intracerebral haemorrhage and traumatic brain injury, and therefore fall under the auspices of neurosurgical management. Nevertheless, the patient should still be seen to promptly.

DOI: 10.1201/9781003493310-9

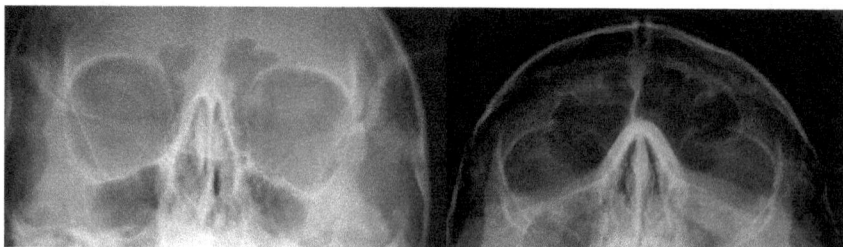

Figure 8.1 Small (left) and large (right) frontal sinus demonstrated on XR.

- OMFS may be asked to attend as part of the formal trauma team in the event of polytrauma; a full OMFS assessment is important in an ATLS approach
  - The team should attend early to introduce themselves, assign roles and receive handover from the pre-hospital team if the patient is brought in by ambulance
  - Ensure the patient is assessed in accordance with ATLS protocol with a primary survey
  - Deal with any other potential injuries in order of priority according to trauma scenario

History

Event

- Preceding events
- Type of event – road traffic accident, fall from height, assault
- Post-event – loss of consciousness, amnesia, seizure

Systems

- Eye – change in vision, loss of vision, double vision, bleeding
- Neurological – headaches, syncope, seizures, loss of consciousness, vomiting
- Nose – nasal trauma – deviation, epistaxis, clear rhinorrhoea

Red flags/Risk factors

- High-impact trauma
- Signs and symptoms of CSF leak, raised intracranial pressure

AMPLE

- Allergies, regular/recent medications, other relevant past medical history, time of last meal

Examination

- General signs of facial fracture – soft tissue bruising, swelling, laceration
- Eye – ocular motility/restriction, pupil size and reaction to light, RAPD
- Frontal bone – indentation or deformity
- Neurology – GCS, cranial nerves, upper and lower limbs

- Skin – supraorbital and supratrochlear paraethesia
- Full set of observations

Management

The principles of managing patients with frontal bone trauma are to aid fracture healing and minimise and manage complications, which may be significant. Outflow tract obstruction is best assessed late (6–12 months) since initial imaging may overstate this due to mucosal swelling, presence of blood and small fragments of bone that will resorb. The need to treat fractures of the posterior wall and the outflow tract is determined by the presence of features that would indicate an increased risk of sinus disease such as mucoceles, or if there is an increased risk of sinus pathogens causing cerebral infection (abscesses, meningitis). Given the multidisciplinary nature of these injuries, all patients should be discussed with neurosurgery, and for outflow tract obstruction an ENT opinion is indicated.

Bedside investigations

- Routine blood tests are rarely indicated
- FBC, U&Es, coagulation profile, group and save/crossmatch can be taken as part of the surgical workup

Imaging

- CT facial bones/Head (Figure 8.2)
  - Assess the anterior wall for any fracture displacement (significant displacement may be considered to be present when the amount of displacement is greater than the width of the bone)
  - Assess posterior wall for presence and degree of displacement
  - Assess nasofrontal outflow tract for patency
- Beta-2 transferrin/tau protein – confirm CSF leak

Medical

- Consider tetanus booster or tranexamic acid if indicated
- IV antibiotics – not usually indicated in closed fractures but may be considered if overlying facial lacerations are present, especially if contaminated
- Analgesia

Conservative management

- Undisplaced and many minimally displaced anterior and posterior wall fractures
- Patent outflow tracts

Surgical management

- Significant visible deformity of anterior wall – ORIF ± coronal flap
- Displaced posterior wall fractures or anterior and posterior wall fractures – cranialization
- Outflow tract obstruction – transnasal procedure

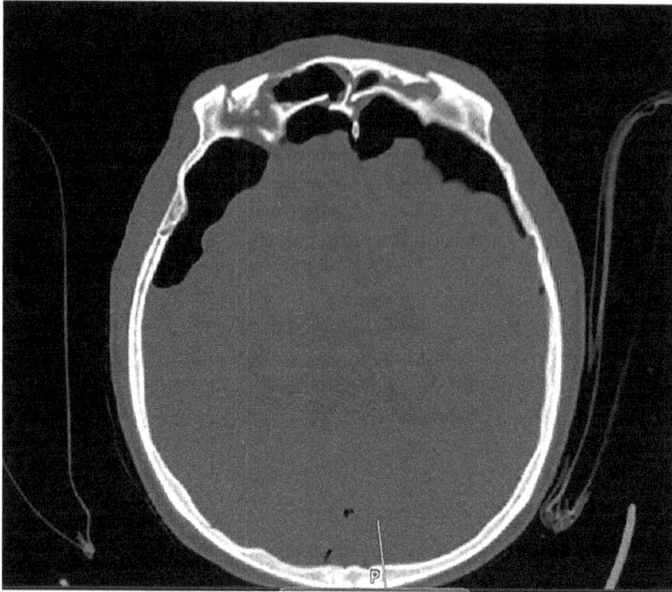

Figure 8.2 Axial CT head demonstrating fractures of anterior and posterior walls of both frontal sinuses with significant displacement and pneumocephalus.

Steps for frontal sinus cranialization

- Coronal flap with pericranial flap separated
- Bifrontal craniotomy
- Dural repair
- Frontal sinus cranialization and mucosa stripping
- Obstruction of frontal outflow tract with bone
- Pericranial flap over outflow tract
- Replacement craniotomy with or without drain placement
- Closure of coronal flap

Discharge and follow-up

- Patients can be discharged once surgical drains have been removed and they are mobile
- Anterior wall fractures – usually 24–48 hours
- Longer following cranialization especially if involved in polytrauma (requires postoperative CT imaging prior to discharge)
- Initial clinic follow-up at 1–2 weeks to review surgical wounds and for signs of infection
- Further follow-up may be arranged at 6–8 weeks
- Anterior wall fractures do not need further follow-up
- Posterior wall fractures are best followed up at 12 months, with new CT imaging
- Outflow tract injuries should be reviewed with a new CT scan at 12 months to confirm patency

MCQs

1) Following a frontal head collision, the presence of which of the following is most likely to indicate a significant frontal fracture?

A) Forehead laceration
B) Clear nasal discharge
C) Epistaxis
D) Nasal congestion
E) Supraorbital paraesthesia

2) What is the main indication for treatment of an isolated fracture of the anterior wall of the frontal sinus?

A) Supraorbital paraesthesia
B) Dural tear
C) Outflow tract obstruction
D) Cosmesis
E) Brow ptosis

3) Which of the following is not a key step in cranialization of the frontal sinus?

A) Exposure of cribriform plate
B) Bifrontal craniotomy
C) Stripping mucosa from anterior wall of sinus
D) Removal of posterior wall of sinus
E) Multilayered coverage of outflow tract

Chapter 9

Facial ballistic trauma
John Breeze

Background

For the purposes of this chapter, wound ballistics refers to the pathology caused by ballistic projectiles, namely low- and high-velocity bullets. Energised fragments from explosive devices are fortunately rarely encountered in civilian practice but can occur in terrorist events and may be sustained by service personnel in conflict or even interpersonal violence.

Although the muzzle velocity of bullets, commonly referred to as low and high velocity, does in part contribute to an understanding of the subsequent injury, it is the energy deposited to the tissues that is more important. The facial region in the body is unique in that it comprises three types of structures that may alter the passage of a projectile, namely the soft tissue, the bony skeleton and the air sinus. For example, a low-velocity projectile that impacts the mandible may shatter it into pieces, but a high-velocity projectile that damages only soft tissue may on occasions produce surprisingly little damage. Projectiles passing through the face often ricochet off the bony skeleton, significantly increasing energy deposition and making it difficult to fully ascertain the injury extent even with three-dimensionally reconstructed imaging.

Potential areas for deterioration

A   damage to the airway from the projectile directly or from swelling in the tissues around it
C   bleeding from major vessels – vascular tissue can be damaged by the temporary cavity of the projectile even if the wound tract itself doesn't go through the vessel

Preparation and equipment

- All ballistic injuries to the face should be treated as OMFS emergencies and the patient must be seen to urgently
- Ensure the patient is in an appropriate high-dependency area with the difficult airway equipment available
- Make a senior colleague aware that you have a ballistic injury
- OMFS may be asked to attend as part of the formal trauma team in the event of polytrauma; a full OMFS assessment is important in an ATLS approach

DOI: 10.1201/9781003493310-10

- The team should attend early to introduce themselves, assign roles and receive handover from the pre-hospital team if the patient is brought in by ambulance
- Ensure the patient is assessed in accordance with ATLS protocol with a primary survey
- Deal with any other potential injuries in order of priority according to trauma scenario

Immediate assessment

- Perform a rapid A to E assessment before proceeding either with immediate resuscitation or taking a history from patient/relative/ambulance crew
- If the patient presents in cardiorespiratory arrest, then commence CPR and resuscitation according to ALS guidelines with the appropriate teams notified
- Many patients will arrive intubated at the scene; if not, early intubation is advisable in the context of potential airway compromise
- Consider escalation to surgical cricothyroidotomy by marking neck landmarks

History

History-taking in a ballistic facial injury should be brief, even if the patient is relatively physiologically stable. An AMPLE history should suffice before proceeding towards examination and, more importantly, a contrast CT. It is often when you are in the position of being able to look at the CT that you come back to complete the history.

Events/Systems

- Preceding events
- Type of event – assault, service personnel conflict, terrorism
- Post-event – blood loss, loss of consciousness, SOB, aspiration/choking, drooling, facial injury

Red flags/Risk factors

- High impact/energy injuries
- Concomitant injury/trauma
- Airway or circulatory compromise

Examination

- General inspection for signs of respiratory distress – noisy breathing (stridor, stertor), tachypnoea, cyanosis, use of accessory muscles, anxiety, agitation, fatigue
- Assess for signs of catastrophic haemorrhage
- Ballistic injury examination
  - Entry and exit wounds (Figure 9.1)
  - Potential wound tract – assume any structure between tracts is damaged
  - Examine from top of scalp to clavicles – scalp lacerations, nasal fractures, facial injury, facial droop, missing teeth, deep damage from small penetrating fragments
  - Neck   haematoma

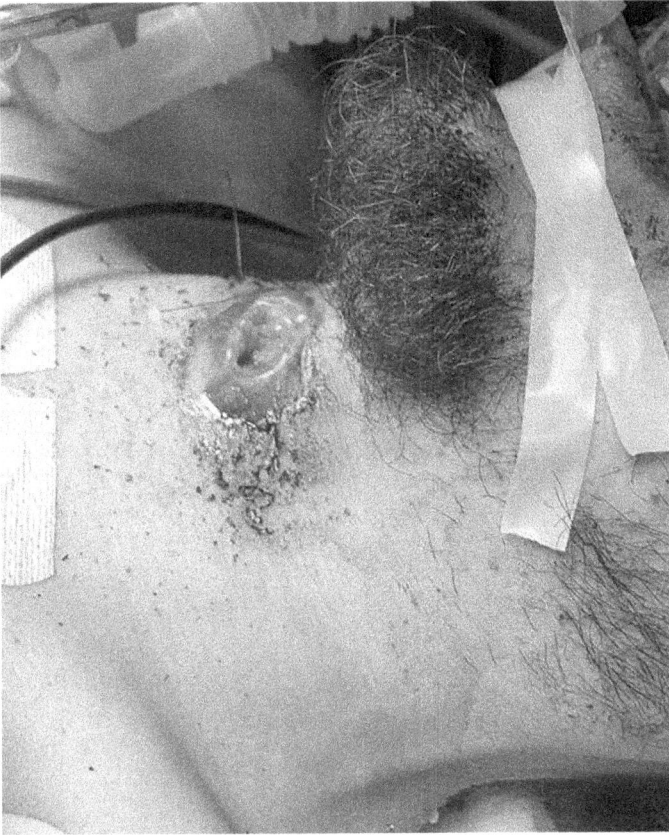

Figure 9.1 Entry gunshot wound into the anterior neck of an intubated patient.

- Full set of observations – assess for signs of respiratory distress (tachypnoea, reduced saturations) or hypovolaemic shock (tachycardia, hypotension)

Management

The principle of management in facial ballistic trauma is to identify the extent of the damage and damage control while minimising complications – namely catastrophic haemorrhage and airway compromise. The key decision from the presentation is regarding immediate surgical exploration (without imaging) versus a more planned approach. Management of these patients often requires an MDT approach with senior OMFS/ENT colleagues, anaesthetics/critical care, ED and radiologists to help guide treatment. The mainstay of management is surgery with a close eye on the airway.

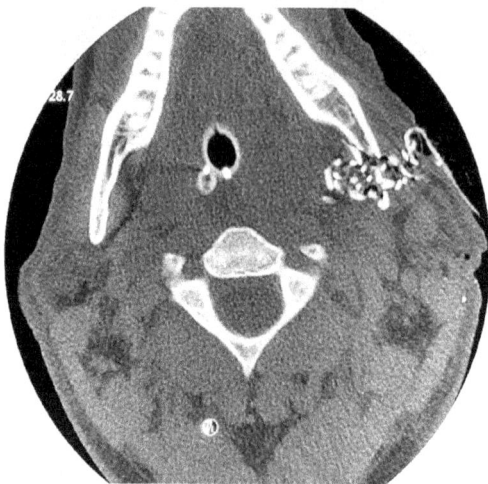

Figure 9.2 Axial CT image showing a gunshot wound to the left mandible with subsequent fracture.

Bedside

- Sit patient up if able
- Oxygenate (15 L high-flow oxygen or high-flow nasal cannula [HFNC] therapy)
- IV tranexamic acid
- Bloods (if able) – FBC, clotting, lactate

Imaging

- CT face and neck with contrast (Figure 9.2) – assess ballistic position if still present and any damage

Surgical

- Clean all soft tissue injuries under general anaesthetic
- Repair any mandible fractures
- Wound exploration and washout
- Surgical tracheostomy is often warranted – allows full examination of the mouth and bringing teeth together for subsequent pan-facial rehabilitation
- NG feeding to allow oral cavity fistulae and any small oesophageal/pharyngeal perforations to heal (that can be missed on CT)

Discharge and follow-up

Ballistic facial injury may result in complex injuries, few of which are often addressed during the initial hospital admission. Injuries can be broadly broken down into soft tissue, bone and teeth. Scarring is not just aesthetically upsetting to the patient; it may limit mouth opening and limit prosthodontic rehabilitation. Although bone injury may warrant augmentation in the longer term, early use of removable prostheses is key, and will allow replacement of damaged teeth. Close working between OMFS and a restorative dentist is essential. Complex defects may require free flap surgery, with the key being to eliminate fistulas, obtain an oral seal and instigate oral feeding as soon as possible. Further reconstructive work may be planned on a semi-elective basis.

Be aware of ...

- The seemingly well patient that is moved out of resus early
- Any delay in obtaining a CT scan, unless the patient is in extremis and requires surgery immediately
- Penetrating airway injury – be aware of possible additional digestive tract injury

MCQs

1) Which of the following best determines the severity of injury in ballistic facial trauma?

   A) The velocity of the projectile
   B) The type of firearm used
   C) The energy deposited into the tissues
   D) The size of the entry wound
   E) The distance from which the projectile was fired

2) In managing a patient with ballistic facial trauma, what is the primary consideration in deciding between immediate surgical exploration and planned surgical intervention?

   A) Presence of soft tissue injury
   B) Extent of airway or circulatory compromise
   C) Size of the entry and exit wounds
   D) Availability of CT imaging
   E) Presence of facial fractures

3) Which of the following is a common long-term consideration in the follow-up of ballistic facial injuries?

   A) Antibiotic prophylaxis for 6 months
   B) Discharge without further reconstructive planning
   C) Immediate dental implants for missing teeth
   D) Avoidance of oral feeding for extended periods
   E) Use of free flap surgery to address complex defects

Chapter 10

Soft tissue injuries
Justin Yeo and Salman Tahir

Background

Craniofacial soft tissue trauma makes up a significant proportion of injuries presenting to the hospital. These injuries can potentially cause significant aesthetic and functional morbidity, especially when there is an associated craniofacial fracture. Loss of tissue with involvement of deeper layers of tissue, and different facial subunits are important considerations because they can make repair and reconstruction challenging. The reconstructive ladder (Figure 10.1) should be consulted when deciding on how best to repair any soft tissue injury. Aesthetic outcome is another important consideration because the face is the most visible part of the body and often has an uneven topography. Injuries should be repaired parallel to the relaxed skin tension lines (RSTL), also known as Langer's lines, to obtain a more cosmetically pleasing outcome, since this will maximise the closure tension.

Potential areas of deterioration

C risk of haemorrhage from open injuries, risk of sepsis from dirty wounds
D risk of disability secondary to head injuries

Preparation and equipment

- This is an OMFS emergency and the patient must be seen to immediately
- OMFS may be asked to attend as part of the formal trauma team in the event of polytrauma; a full OMFS assessment is important in an ATLS approach
  - The team should attend early to introduce themselves, assign roles and receive handover from the pre-hospital team if the patient is brought in by ambulance
  - Ensure the patient is assessed in accordance with ATLS protocol with a primary survey
  - Deal with any other potential injuries in order of priority according to trauma scenario
- Attend with local anaesthesia, suture pack, saline for irrigation, sutures of your choice (preferably vicryl for deeper layers, Prolene/Ethilon for skin)

DOI: 10.1201/9781003493310-11

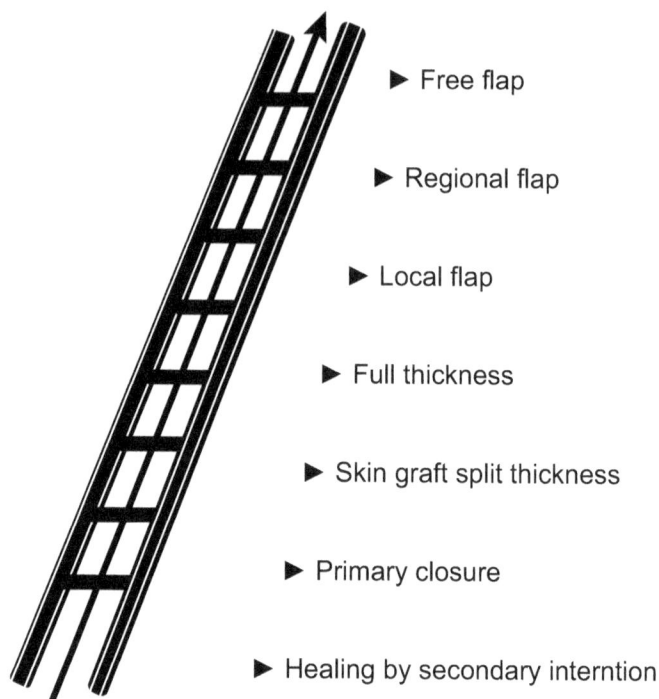

Figure 10.1 Reconstructive ladder.

History

Events

- Preceding events
- Type of event – assault, road traffic accident, fall, self-harm, clean vs dirty
- Post-event – impaired function (sensory/motor changes), blood loss

Systems

- Ears – otalgia, otorrhoea (bloody, clear), hearing loss, facial weakness, vertigo
- Eyes – vision changes, increasing pain/pressure, colour changes
- Neurological – vomiting, amnesia, headaches, syncope, seizures
- Nose – clear rhinorrhoea, epistaxis, septal deviation, septal haematoma
- Oral – teeth mobility/avulsion, mobility of maxilla/mandible, change in bite, numbness/weakness of lower lip, numbness of upper lip/maxillary teeth, swallowing change
- Voice – change in voice

Red flags/Risk factors

- High-impact trauma
- Significant tissue loss
- Active bleeding
- Injuries to important structures of face – eyes, nose, ears, mouth

AMPLE

- Allergies, regular/recent medication, relevant past medical history, time of last meal

Examination

- General inspection – active bleeding, weapon in situ, patient's consciousness level
- Open wound (Figure 10.2) – size, depth, soft tissue loss, viability of wound edges, structures exposed, level of contamination
- Closed wound – ecchymosis, deformity, swelling
- Ophthalmology – visual acuity, eye movements, periorbital haematoma/ecchymosis, subconjunctival haemorrhage, fluorescein dye for corneal abrasions, involvement of medial/lateral canthus
- Neurology – cranial nerve examination, upper and lower limb examination, GCS
- Otoscopy – tympanic membrane perforation, haemotympanum, EAC fracture, otorrhoea (bloody vs clear), exposed cartilage
- Rhinology – septal haematoma, deviation, exposed cartilage, epistaxis
- Parotid gland – suspect if injury between pretragal region to middle half of ipsilateral upper lip
- Full set of observations

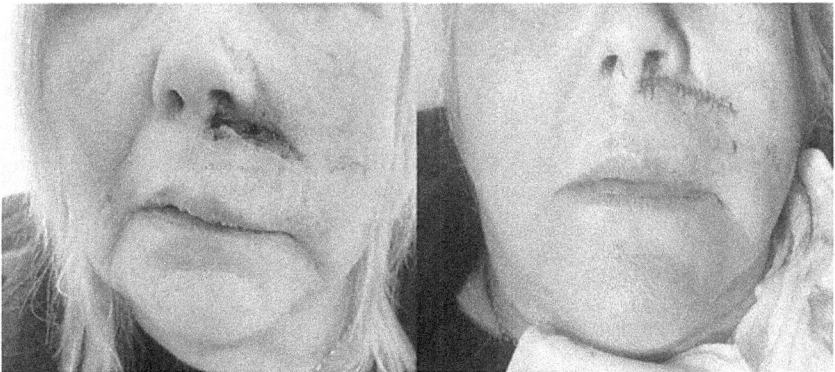

Figure 10.2 Soft tissue injury of the left subnasale before (left) and after (right) closure.

Management

The principle of managing patients with soft tissue injuries is based on the reconstructive ladder and considering whether the wound is clean vs dirty. Minimal tension closure should be achieved, with debridement of any non-viable tissue before closure. Form and function should be prioritised, followed by aesthetic considerations. If injuries are complex and involve other facial organs or if patients are unable to tolerate local anaesthesia (paediatric patients), consider repair under general anaesthesia. The earlier isolated soft tissue injuries are repaired, the better the postoperative aesthetic results. Delays increase the risk of infection and obscures landmarks, due to swelling, which will negatively affect the outcome. If available, consider obtaining clinical photographs of the injuries before and after repair. The main principles in suture technique are equal distribution of tension in the deeper layers, eversion of wound edges and minimal trauma when handling tissue.

Bedside investigations

- Blood tests – FBC, coagulation screen, group and save/crossmatch if injuries are significant, or concerns about bleeding or haemostasis
- Wound swab – if actively infected

General

- Consider tetanus booster if dirty injury
- Safeguarding concerns (especially in paediatrics) if injury does not fit history

Isolated soft tissue injury

- Assess and repair as soon as possible
- Wash out (saline, chlorhexidine, povidone iodine) if dirty wound; saline or sterile water wash in eyes is preferred (neutral pH)
- LA infiltration (+ adrenaline to help with haemostasis)
- Repair using reconstructive ladder
- Debride non-viable wound edges
- Each layer should be closed in turn (muscle/cartilage, subcutaneous tissue, skin)

Discharge and follow-up

- Discharge from hospital once successfully repaired (assuming no other injuries)
- Consider topical or oral antibiotics (5–7 days) if high risk of infection (immunosuppressed patient, dirty wound) or complex injury
- For most cases which are repaired primarily, follow-up with GP for suture removal or emergency clinic in 7–10 days

MCQs

1) You've been called to see a 21-year-old female in A&E resus about a forehead laceration. She was involved in a road traffic accident in which the driver was killed on-site. What is the most important investigation you should review before attending to this patient?

   A) Up-to-date bloods
   B) Trauma CT
   C) Past medical history
   D) Medications that have been given so far
   E) None – attend to the patient immediately

2) You've been called to emergency theatres to close a lip laceration for a 3-year-old under general anaesthesia. The lip laceration crosses the vermillion border and extends down to orbicularis oris. In which order will you carry out the repair?

   I. Repair skin layers
   II. Holding stitch to align the vermillion border
   III. Repair the muscle layers
   IV. Local anaesthesia infiltration

   A) III, I, II, IV
   B) IV, III, II, I
   C) III, II, I, IV
   D) II, III, IV, I
   E) III, IV, II, I

3) In which of these cases would you consider using adjuncts (glue, steri-strips, staples) for closure rather than sutures?

   A) Forehead laceration in 2 year old
   B) Singular cat bite puncture wound in cheek of a 7 year old
   C) Superficial lip laceration in 5 year old crossing vermillion border
   D) Superficial laceration of nasal alar rim in 36 year old
   E) Cheek abrasion in 79 year old patient who fell

Chapter 11

TMJ dislocation

David McGoldrick

Background

The temporomandibular joint is composed of the condyle of the mandible and the glenoid fossa of the temporal bone. A fibrocartilage disc lies between the bony surfaces and aids in function. Three dense ligaments – the sphenomandibular, stylomandibular and lateral ligaments – support the joint. Dislocations may be unilateral or bilateral and may occur in an anterior, lateral, superior or posterior direction. Anterior dislocations, when the condyle lies anterior to the articular eminence of the temporal bone, are by far the most common and may be due to traumatic or non-traumatic causes (Figure 11.1). Activities associated with over-opening of the mandible are commonly implicated and include yawning, laughing and procedures such as dental treatment or general anaesthesia. Dislocations in other directions are rarer and more likely to be associated with trauma, possible fractures and damage to adjacent structures. Treatment is focused at early reduction of the dislocation with closed methods. Occasionally, adjuncts such as sedation or anaesthesia are required to assist in this.

History

Symptoms

- Onset, time since event
- Laterality
- Precipitating event – extreme mouth opening, trauma, dental treatment, surgery
- History of previous dislocations
- Previous operations/trauma/treatment

Systems

- Airway – drooling
- Ear – otorrhoea, hearing loss
- Neurological – cranial nerve palsy, seizures
- Voice – change in speech (due to being locked open)

DOI: 10.1201/9781003493310-12

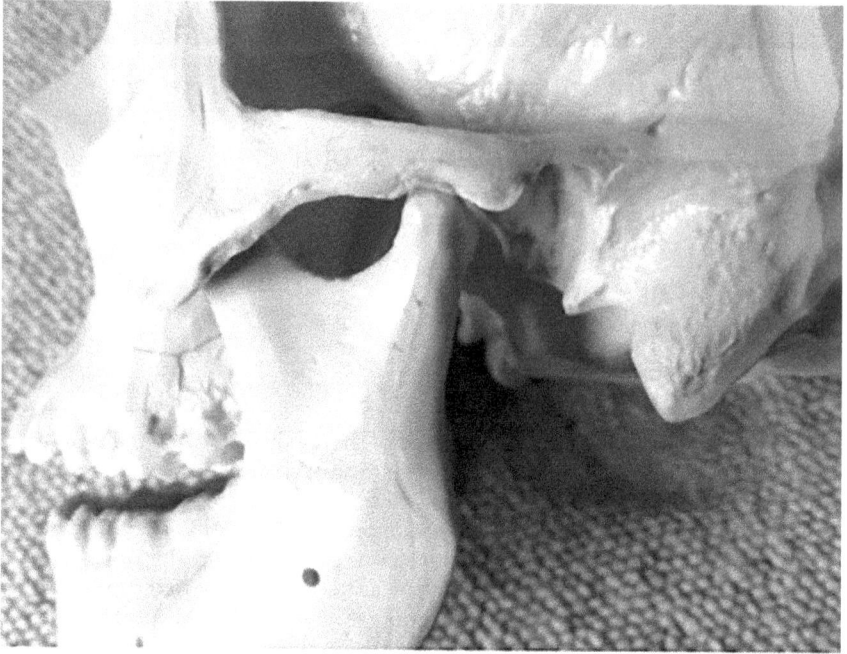

Figure 11.1 Model demonstration of left anterior TMJ dislocation.

Past medical history

- Connective tissue disease
- Neurological or neurodegenerative disease
- Rheumatological disease
- Previous surgery

Social history

- Smoking, alcohol status
- Nutritional status

Examination

- General inspection – nutritional status, difficult speech, drooling
- Intraoral
    - Usually locked open
    - Dental occlusion
    - Bite – anterior open bite if bilateral, ipsilateral lateral open bite if unilateral
- Extraoral
    - Depression in pre-auricular region
    - Signs of trauma
    - Chin point may be deviated to contralateral side if unilateral dislocation
- Cranial nerves – especially V, VII, VIII

Management

The principles of management are focused on prompt closed reduction of the dislocation. Prolonged dislocation will increase muscle spasm and potentially make reduction more difficult. Infiltration of local anaesthesia may be considered for pain control and to aid with the reduction. In difficult cases or cases with a delayed presentation, consideration should be given to the use of sedation or general anaesthesia.

Imaging

- Usually not required
- OPG – can confirm position of condyle outside fossa and assess for possible associated fractures
- CT – may be useful in dislocations other than anterior or with concomitant fractures

Closed reduction

- Bimanual method – most commonly used
  - Downward and backward pressure placed on posterior mandible intra-orally
- External method – external pressure to allow sequential reduction
- Gag method – stimulation of gag reflex but may cause vomiting

Recurrent dislocation

- Non-surgical
  - Botulinum toxin injections
  - Intra-articular injections

- Surgical
  - Usually focuses on augmenting or removing the articular eminence

Discharge and follow-up

- Simple acute dislocation – discharge with advice (avoid wide mouth opening, soft diet)
- Circumferential head-chin bandage can minimise mouth opening
- Consider follow-up if risk factors or recurrent dislocation are present

Red flags

- Significant delay in presentation
- Superior/posterior/lateral dislocations potentially associated with fractures and damage to adjacent structures

When to refer from primary care

- Any suspected dislocation should be referred for prompt assessment and reduction to the local ED/OMFS department

Risk factors for TMJ dislocation

- Anatomic mismatch between the fossa and articular eminence
- Temporomandibular ligament or capsule weakness
- Connective tissue disorders (e.g., Ehlers–Danlos or Marfan syndrome)
- Previous dislocation
- Torn ligaments

MCQs

1) In which direction does TMJ dislocation normally occur?

    A) Anterior
    B) Posterior
    C) Medial
    D) Lateral
    E) Superior

2) Which is the most commonly used method for closed reduction in TMJ dislocations?

    A) External method
    B) Gag method
    C) Bimanual method
    D) Botulinum toxin injection
    E) Intra-articular injection

3) Following reduction, which of the following is usually implemented?

    A) Circumferential head-chin bandage
    B) Immobilisation with intermaxillary fixation (IMF)
    C) Nasogastric tube feeding
    D) Tracheostomy
    E) Inpatient stay until eating as normal

Neck haematoma

Farhan Khalid and Prav Praveen

Background

A haematoma is the collection of congealed blood in tissue, organ or body space and usually results from broken larger blood vessels damaged at the time of operation or any injury. In contrast, bruising is damage to smaller blood vessels and appears as blue and/or purple discolouration which changes colour upon healing. A postoperative neck haematoma is a serious complication of head and neck surgery necessitating immediate assessment and prompt management. It usually occurs due to slippage of ligature of a prominent neck vessel in the postoperative period, or rarely a generalised ooze which is difficult to control intra-operatively. Meticulous tissue dissection, vessel control and haemostasis are key to preventing a postoperative neck haematoma. A postoperative neck haematoma in free flap reconstruction of patients poses a risk to flap blood supply (pedicle) leading to congestion and obstruction of venous drainage and consequently arterial compromise and flap failure.

Potential areas for deterioration

A airway compromise due to expanding neck haematoma in a patient without tracheostomy
B difficulty in breathing due to compromised air exchange potentially due to haematoma shifting the trachea to the contralateral side
C risk of hypovolaemic shock if large active bleeding
E free flap compromise due to expanding neck haematoma

Preparation and equipment

- This is an OMFS emergency, and the patient should be seen to immediately
- Attend with difficult airway trolley, headlight, suture/staple remover, suction, high-flow oxygen
- Escalate to a senior OMFS/ENT clinician and anaesthetist

DOI: 10.1201/9781003493310-13

History

Symptoms – pain, swelling

- Onset, duration, progression
- Better or worse
- Exacerbating or relieving factors
- Operative details – what procedure, indication, any other perioperative complications, abnormal anatomy, documentation of recurrent laryngeal nerve preservation, method of wound closure

Systems

- Airway – difficulty in breathing, SOB, aspiration/choking, drooling
- Oesophagus – dysphagia, odynophagia, regurgitation
- Voice – change in voice

Risk factors/Red flags

- Known coagulopathy
- Long procedure with intraoperative complications
- Obesity

AMPLE

- Allergies, regular/recent medications, other relevant past medical history, time of last meal

Examination

- General inspection – patient positioning, agitation, anxiety, respiratory distress, stridor
- Wound – dehiscence, discharge, erythema
- Neck – palpate around wound to assess for swelling (fluctuant, boggy, hard, tender), range of motion, torticollis (Figure 12.1)
- Drain – output, haematoma can still form in the presence of drains
- Full set of observations – assess for signs of respiratory distress (desaturation, tachypnoea)

Management

The principle of management in patients with a neck haematoma is early recognition and rapid evacuation of the haematoma to prevent airway compression and free flap compromise. The following management steps suggest a stepwise approach. If the patient has improved and is stable after each step, then consider a planned return to theatre after discussion with the senior surgeon and anaesthetist.

Initial management

- High-flow oxygen (15 L/min through a non-rebreather mask)
- Head-up nursing
- Reassure and calm the patient

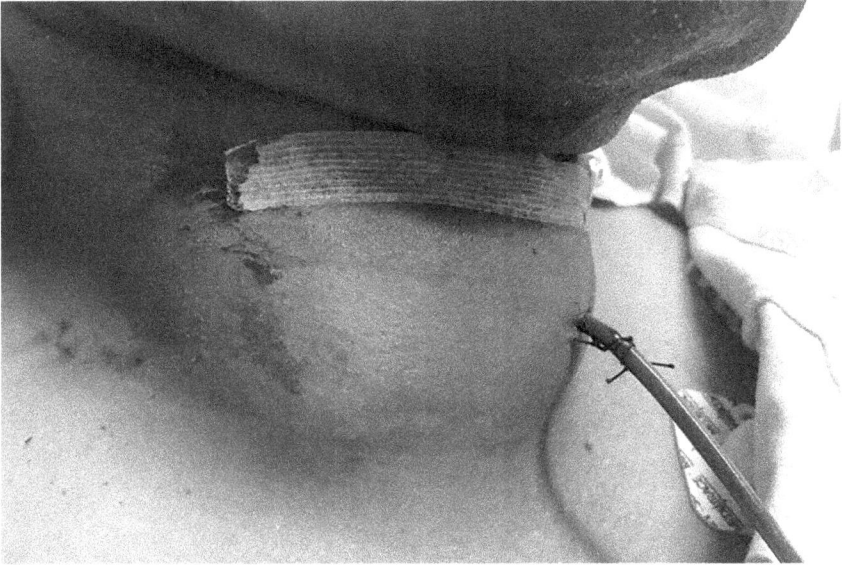

Figure 12.1 Neck haematoma in a patient with a surgical drain.

- Stop feed/keep NBM
- Ensure bloods including group and save and crossmatch are available
- Medical adjuncts – consider IV corticosteroid, IV tranexamic acid
- Release of neck staples/sutures if rapid expanding haematoma and imminent airway risk

Return to theatre

- Consent – for exploration, evacuation of haematoma ± definite airway (if no pre-existing tracheostomy), explanation of benefits, risks and alternatives
- Stable patients – return to theatre urgently after consent and planning for safe intubation and surgical approach
- Unstable patients (impending airway compromise) – immediate intubation with anaesthetics following bedside haematoma release, prepare for FONA
- Surgical management – haematoma evacuation, wash, stopping any bleeding vessels (cautery, ties, clips)
- Consider insertion of a suction drain

Discharge and follow-up

- Discharge patients if they have been stable for 24–48 hours with no signs of haematoma recollection or other postoperative complications
- Follow up according to surgical preoperative plan

MCQs

1) What is the most common cause of neck haematoma?

   A) Patient comorbidities
   B) Obesity
   C) Smoking
   D) Slippage of ligature and generalised ooze
   E) Smoking

2) What is the key step in managing neck haematoma following surgery or trauma?

   A) Check bloods
   B) Check clotting
   C) Assess and manage airway
   D) Reassurance of patient
   E) Consider ultrasound

3) What is the appropriate management of an expanding neck haematoma following head and neck reconstruction surgery?

   A) Reassurance of the patient
   B) Check bloods
   C) Arrange group and save
   D) Exploration of neck and evacuation of haematoma
   E) Close monitoring

Chapter 13

Free flap compromise
Farhan Khalid and Sat Parmar

Background

Free flaps are considered at the top of the reconstruction ladder and can either be soft tissue or composite (bone and soft tissue) harvested from different body parts with their respective blood supply (pedicle) and anastomosed to recipient vessels, close to the area being reconstructed. They are commonly used for reconstruction following ablative surgery but can be used for other reasons such as osteoradionecrosis of the jaw, major trauma and tissue loss or correction of congenital deformities. The advantages of free flap reconstruction is its own blood supply, availability of various tissues to match the defect and versatility to provide better cosmetic and functional outcomes. Free flap reconstruction following head and neck ablative surgery is the gold standard, aiming to preserve and improve form and function of oro-facial defects.

Examples of head and neck free flaps and their pedicles

Soft tissue flaps

- Radial forearm free flap based on radial artery
- Anterolateral thigh flap – circumflex femoral artery
- Lateral arm free flap – posterior radial collateral artery
- Latissimus dorsi muscle flap – thoracodorsal artery
- Rectus abdominis flap – deep inferior epigastric artery

Composite flaps

- Fibula flap – peroneal artery
- Iliac bone flap (DCIA) – deep circumflex iliac artery
- Scapula bone flap – circumflex scapular artery

Potential areas for deterioration

A airway compromise
C risk of septic shock in infected cases of flap compromise

DOI: 10.1201/9781003493310-14

Preparation and equipment

- This is an OMFS emergency and the patient should be seen to immediately
- Attend with a headlight/torch, wooden spatula, lubricating jelly and a hand-held Doppler

History

Symptoms – swelling/pain

- Onset, timing and duration
- Better or worse
- Preceding symptoms – pressure, pain, swelling

Systems

- Airway – difficulty in breathing, SOB, drooling
- Oesophagus – dysphagia, odynophagia
- Voice – change in voice (depending on flap position and presence of tracheostomy)

Risk factors/Red flags

- Patient factors
  - Coagulopathy
  - Obesity
  - Smoking
  - Previous radiotherapy

- Operative factors
  - Poor quality vessels
  - Technical errors
  - Postoperative infection

AMPLE

- Allergies, regular/recent medications, other relevant past medical history, time of last meal

Examination

- General inspection – stable or unstable, patient posture
- Respiratory distress – noisy breathing (stridor, stertor), tachypnoea, cyanosis, use of accessory muscles, anxiety, agitation, fatigue
- Voice – speaking in full sentences, quality of voice
- Neck – range of motion, torticollis, swelling
- Flap (Figures 13.1 and 13.2)
  - Inspection – swelling, colour (pink, pale, white, blue tinge), expanding
  - Palpation – capillary refill, temperature, consistency (soft, firm, boggy), turgor
  - Scratch test – delayed, no blood, dark blood (should be done by a senior clinician)
  - Special tests – handheld or implantable Doppler (pulsation sound – arterial/venous, good, weak, no sounds)

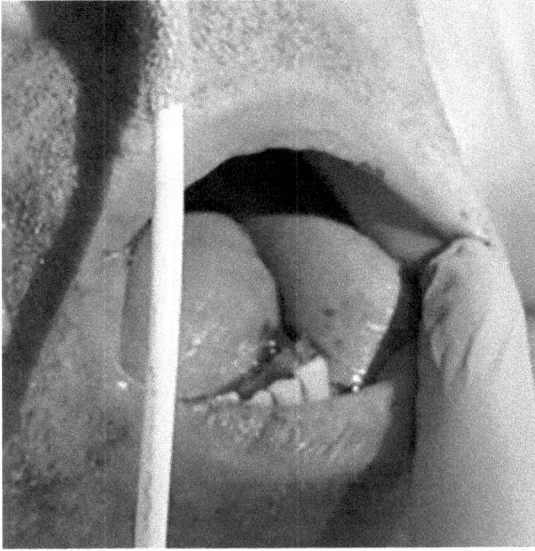

Figure 13.1 Venous compromise of the free flap reconstructing the defect left mandible.

Management

The principle of management in patients with free flap compromise is rapid assessment and decision regarding management to maximise the chance of flap salvage. If left unrecognised and untreated, there can be gradual deterioration of flap perfusion leading to flap necrosis, failure, sepsis and potential risk to airway (depending upon flap location / area of reconstruction and presence of pre-existing tracheostomy). In cases of flap compromise, the mainstay of management is surgical. It is essential to recognise free flap blood flow compromise in order to salvage free flap reconstruction and prevent subsequent morbidity to the patient.

Bedside investigations

- Reassess flap in half an hour if not sure about flap compromise with repeat Doppler
- Seek senior advice

Surgery

- Once diagnosis confirmed or high suspicion of flap compromise
- Keep the patient NBM
- Consent the patient by explaining benefits, risks and alternatives
- Inform anaesthetist (if no tracheostomy then airway management can be challenging)
- Involve MDT to enable holistic surgical planning, patient preparation and utilisation of resources

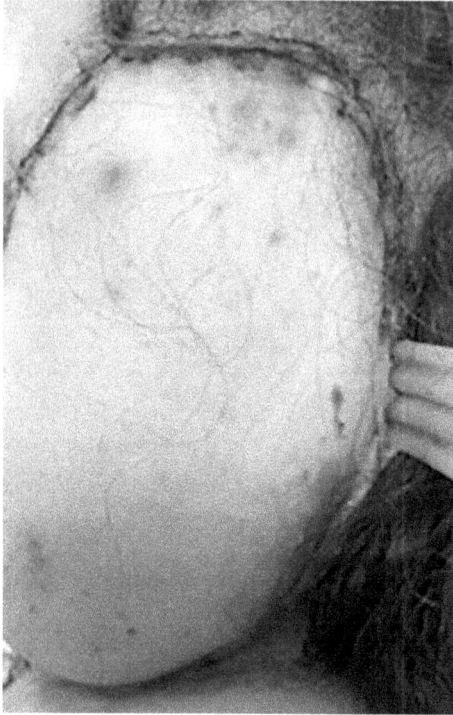

Figure 13.2 Arterial compromise with pale flap with loss of Doppler signal and no blood on scratch testing.

Table 13.1 Signs of Arterial and Venous Compromise

Assessment	Arterial Compromise	Venous Compromise
Flap colour	Pale or mottled	Cyanotic, bluish or dusky
Capillary refill	Sluggish (>2 seconds) or no refill	Brisk (<1 sec)
Tissue turgor	Flat, turgor decreased	Tense, turgor increased
Doppler signals	Absence of pulsatile arterial signal	Absence of continuous venous signal
Scratch test	Scant or no dark blood	Rapid bleeding of dark blood

MCQs

1) What is the gold standard treatment for reconstruction of an oro-facial defect?

   A) Pedicled flap
   B) Skin grafting
   C) Local flap
   D) Free flaps
   E) Healing by secondary intention

2) What is the primary aim for reconstruction of an oral cavity defect following oncological resection?

   A) Improve lip seal
   B) Prevent contraction
   C) Improve form, function and aesthetics
   D) Prevent scarring
   E) Improve speech

3) What is the sign of venous failure in free flap reconstructions?

   A) Pale flap
   B) Soft flap
   C) Bluish flap
   D) Rigid flap
   E) Capillary refill >3 seconds

4) What is the sign of arterial failure in free flap reconstructions?

   A) Bluish flap
   B) Pale flap
   C) Rigid flap
   D) Good Doppler signal
   E) Capillary refill 1–2 seconds

5) What is the usual protocol for free flap monitoring?

   A) Ultrasound scan
   B) Clinical assessment
   C) Specialist test
   D) Blood tests
   E) Imaging

Section II

Elective

Oral cavity malignancy

David McGoldrick

Background

Approximately 300,000–400,000 cases of oral cavity malignancy are reported worldwide annually. Incidence varies by region with the disease being one of the most common cancers in parts of Asia but only the sixteenth most common cancer in the UK. The vast majority of cases (>90%) are caused by squamous cell carcinoma, with smoking and alcohol representing the most common risk factors. A synergistic effect exists when both of these risk factors are present. Betel nut use, common in Asian populations, is a further significant risk factor. A number of pre-malignant conditions also exist which carry a risk of transformation to oral cancer. The majority of patients are male with an average age of 65 years. Although the oral cavity is a site easily accessible for examination, many cases present at an advanced stage. Workup involves tissue diagnosis and cross-sectional imaging for staging. Curative treatment is primarily surgical with adjuvant radiotherapy or chemoradiotherapy dependent on histology.

Variable presenting symptoms of oral cavity malignancy

- A persistent non-healing mouth ulcer (>3 weeks)
- A persistent oral swelling (>3 weeks)
- A red or white patch
- Unexplained tooth mobility
- Non-healing extraction socket
- Altered sensation in the facial region
- Persistent neck mass (>3 weeks)
- Otalgia
- Obstructive symptoms – respiratory distress
- Constitutional symptoms – unexplained weight loss, malnutrition, fever or night sweats

History

Symptoms – may be variable

- Onset, timing and duration
- Laterality (if neck lump/pain or oral cavity lesion)
- Better or worse
- Preceding lesion

DOI: 10.1201/9781003493310-16

Systems

- Airway – SOB, aspiration/choking, drooling
- Neurological – loss of consciousness, seizure
- Oesophagus – dysphagia, odynophagia
- Voice – slurring of speech
- Systemic – unexplained persistent fever, weight loss, malnutrition, night sweats, reduced appetite

Past medical history

- States of immunocompromise
- Previous malignancy and treatment (especially radiotherapy)

Social history

- Smoking, alcohol status
- Nutritional status
- Performance status
- Impact on quality of life and occupation, activities of daily living and hobbies

Examination

- General inspection – nutritional status, signs of respiratory distress
- Oral cavity (Figures 14.1 and 14.2)
  - Extent of lesion
  - Hard and soft palate
  - Invasion of adjacent structures
  - Altered sensation of lip/tongue
  - Tongue mobility
  - Tooth mobility and dental assessment
- Neck – regional lymphadenopathy
- Extremities – assess sites of potential free flap harvest: skin quality, prior surgery, vascular assessment
- FNE – rule out synchronous primaries of head and neck, allows assessment of tongue base if concern for extension to that site, assess airway (usually performed by ENT)

Management

The principle of management for patients with head and neck malignancy is a shared management plan with the MDT taking into account patient wishes. Careful discussion and counselling of patients is essential since primary (chemo) radiotherapy and/or surgical resection may result in significant changes in the patient's quality of life. Initial workup includes staging investigations and histological confirmation with a representative biopsy of the lesion. Inflammation from a biopsy may distort imaging interpretation and consideration should be given to performing imaging prior to biopsy provided treatment is not delayed as a result. Surgery remains the primary treatment modality in oral cancer. This is often combined with adjuvant radiotherapy ± chemotherapy based on definitive histology. Radiotherapy may be considered in those unfit for surgery but may carry

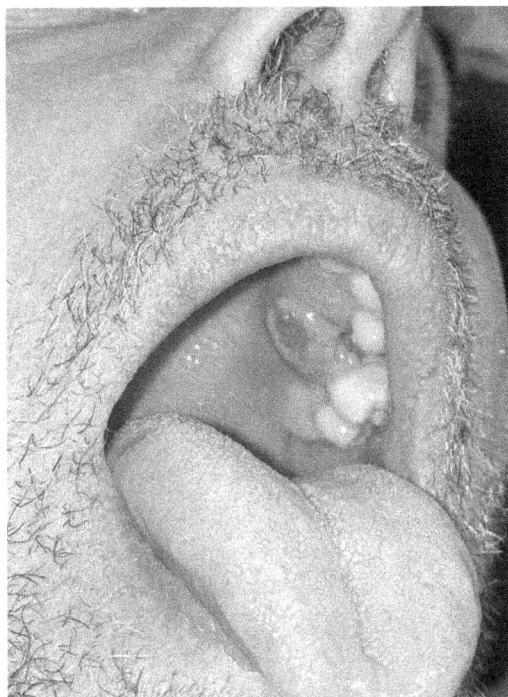

Figure 14.1 Hard palate SCC.

significant morbidity. Palliative treatment may be considered in patients presenting with very advanced disease or in those of low performance status.

Bedside tests

- Bloods and ECG – may be employed for a baseline status

Imaging

- CT neck and thorax
  - Radiological staging of the primary site
  - Cervical lymph node involvement
  - Metastatic disease
  - Bony invasion
- US neck + FNAC/core biopsy – cervical node involvement
- MRI neck – detailed assessment of soft tissue tumour extent or medullary bony invasion
- PET/CT – recommended in N3 disease
- OPG – dental assessment (Figure 14.3)

Histological diagnosis

- Essential to confirm diagnosis (usually under local anaesthetic in clinic)

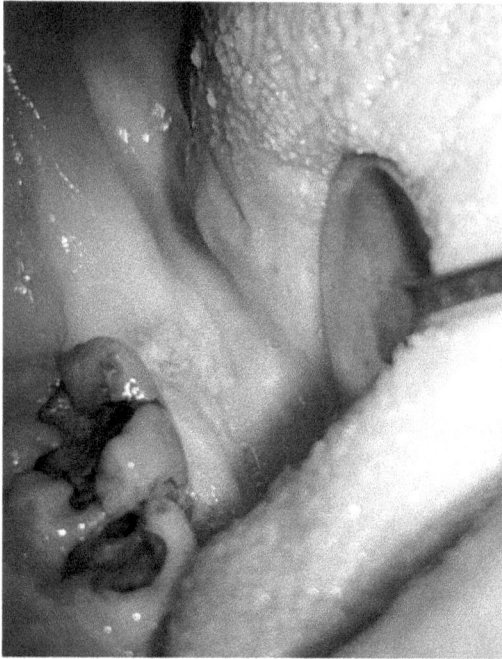

Figure 14.2 Retromolar area SCC.

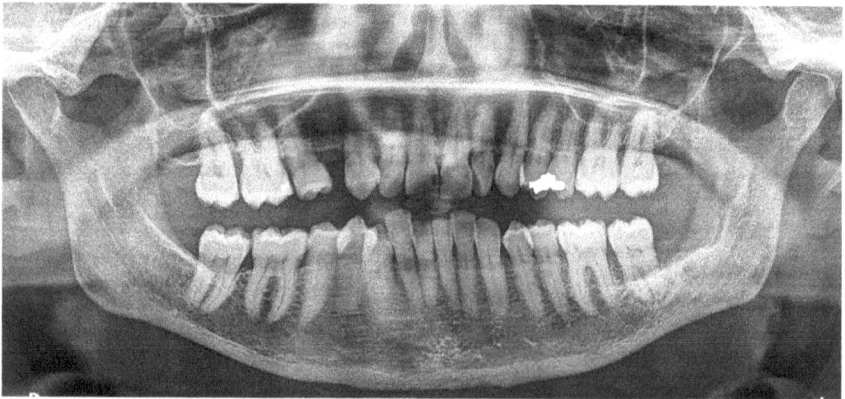

Figure 14.3 OPG demonstrating bony invasion from left oral cavity SCC.

Early-stage disease (T1/T2)

- Primary site – surgery ± reconstruction (Figure 14.4)
- Neck – elective neck dissection or SLNB if N0; therapeutic neck dissection if N+
- Adjuvant treatment – radiotherapy or chemoradiotherapy dependent on histology

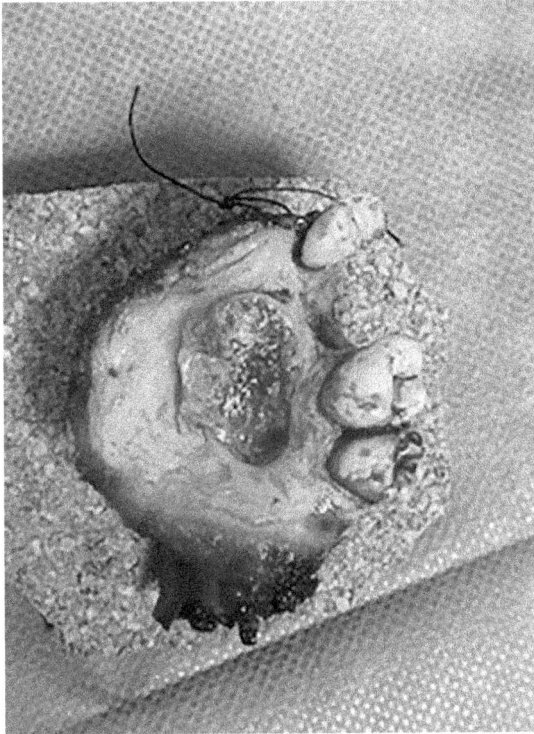

Figure 14.4 Hard palate SCC following surgical resection.

Table 14.1 Primary Tumour Staging for Oral Cavity Malignancy

Tx	Primary tumour cannot be assessed
T0	No evidence of primary tumour
Tis	Carcinoma in situ
T1	Tumour ≤2 cm and DOI ≤5 mm
T2	Tumour ≤2 cm and DOI >5 mm and ≤10 mm Or tumour >2 cm but ≤4 cm and DOI ≤10 mm
T3	Tumour >4 cm Or any DOI >10 m
T4a	Tumour >4 cm and DOI >10 mm Or tumour invades through cortical bone of mandible, maxillary sinus or invades skin of the face
T4b	Tumour invades masticator space, pterygoid plates or skull base and/or encases internal carotid artery

Source: From the UICC TNM 8th Edition.

Advanced-stage disease (T3/T4)

- Primary site – surgery ± reconstruction
- Neck – elective or therapeutic neck dissection
- Adjuvant treatment – radiotherapy or chemoradiotherapy dependent on histology

Recurrent disease

- Salvage surgery
- Radiotherapy
- Palliation

Discharge and follow-up

Regular clinical follow-up is recommended for a minimum of 5 years. After this time the risk of recurrence is low, but patients or clinicians may wish to continue surveillance. Patient-initiated review is encouraged since most recurrences will present symptomatically. A common review schedule is as follows:

- Years 1–2 – every 2 months
- Years 3–4 – every 3–4 months
- Year 5 – every 6 months
- >5 years – annually

When to refer from primary care

- A persistent non-healing mouth ulcer (>3 weeks)
- A persistent oral swelling (>3 weeks)
- A red or white patch
- A persistent neck lump (>3 weeks)

Indications for adjuvant radiotherapy

- Close margins
- T3/T4 disease
- Node positive
- Perineural invasion
- Lymphovascular invasion

Indications for adjuvant chemotherapy

- Extranodal extension
- Positive margins

Members of the MDT closely involved in the management of head and neck malignancy

- Maxillofacial and plastic surgery
- Otolaryngology
- Oncology

- Dentist
- Palliative care team
- Anaesthetics
- Radiology
- Histopathology
- Dietician
- Speech and language therapy
- Head and neck cancer nurse specialist
- Physiotherapist and occupational therapist
- Community support teams – GP, Macmillan cancer support, district nurses, psychologist

Adverse effects of radiotherapy

- Pain
- Skin erythema
- Mucositis
- Fibrosis and scarring of head and neck structures
- Dysphagia
- Lymphoedema
- Stiffness of jaw, neck and shoulders

MCQs

1) Which of the following would be most concerning for an oral cavity malignancy?

   A) Persistent non-healing ulcer
   B) Change in voice
   C) Neck lump
   D) Restricted neck range of motion
   E) Trismus

2) What is commonly used as first-line treatment in oral cavity malignancy?

   A) Chemotherapy
   B) Radiotherapy
   C) Chemoradiotherapy
   D) Immunotherapy
   E) Surgery

3) What is the minimum follow-up usually required for patients with oral cavity malignancies?

   A) 1 year
   B) 2 years
   C) 3 years
   D) 5 years
   E) 10 years

Chapter 15

Cutaneous malignancy

Ashwin Kerai

Background

The three most common skin cancers are basal cell carcinoma (BCC), cutaneous squamous cell carcinoma (cSCC) and cutaneous malignant melanoma. The incidences of all three types are increasing and are directly related to ultraviolet (UV) light exposure. BCCs are slow growing, locally invasive and destructive keratinocyte cancer. It is the most common form of cancer. cSCC is derived from the cells within the epidermis that make keratin. It is an invasive disease and has a propensity to metastasize to regional and distant sites. Malignant melanoma is an aggressive skin cancer in which there is uncontrolled growth of melanocytes. The management of cutaneous melanoma is rapidly developing with the emergence of immunotherapy agents.

History

Symptoms – variable and depends on the subtype – cSCC tends to be more aggressive and symptomatic

- Onset, duration and progression
- Location
- Pain, itching, bleeding or ulceration
- Scabbing (classic feature of BCC)
- Single or multiple
- Change – size, colour

Systems

- Neck – parotid or neck lymphadenopathy
- Systematic – weight loss, B symptoms

Red flags/Risk factors

- Rapid increase in size
- Excessive UV exposure (e.g., sunbed use)
- Fitzpatrick skin type 1 and 2
- Large number of naevi

DOI: 10.1201/9781003493310-17

Past medical history

- Previous skin cancer
- States of immunocompromise (especially solid organ transplant recipients)
- Anticoagulant use
- Previous skin burns/sunburns
- Strong family history of skin cancer
- Genetic conditions – xeroderma pigmentosum, Gorlin–Goltz syndrome, familial atypical multiple mole melanoma (FAMMM) syndrome, Rombo syndrome, atypical or dysplastic naevus syndrome

Drug history

- Allergies

Social history

- Occupation (particularly outdoor workers with sun exposure)
- Smoking, alcohol status
- Nutrional status
- Performance status
- Hobbies (particularly outdoor with sun exposure)
- Previous history of living in countries with high sun exposure
- Impact on quality of life, activities of daily living and hobbies

Examination

- Fitzpatrick skin type (Table 15.1)
- Examine the lesion in good light with magnification
- Pigmented lesions (Figures 15.1 and 15.2)
  - ABCDE characteristics
    - Asymmetry, border irregularity, colour variation, diameter >6 mm, evolving
  - Glasgow 7-point checklist (Table 15.2)
  - Clinical features (Table 15.3)

Table 15.1 Fitzpatrick Skin Type

Skin Type	Typical Features	Tanning Ability
I	Pale white skin, blue/green eyes, blonde/red hair	Always burns, does not tan
II	Fair skin, blue eyes	Burns easily, tans poorly
III	Darker white skin	Tans after initial burn
IV	Light brown skin	Burns minimally, tans easily
V	Brown skin	Rarely burns, tans darkly easily
VI	Dark brown or black skin	Never burns, always tans darkly

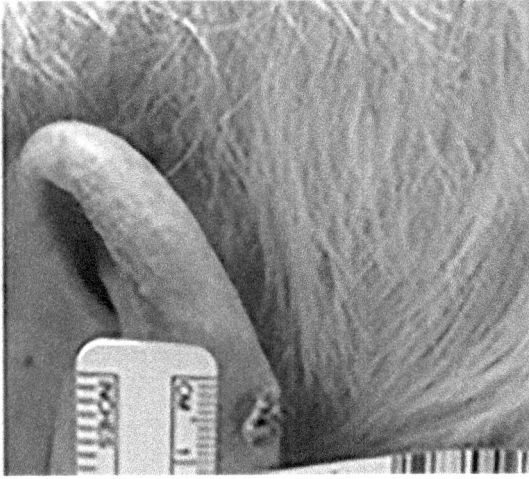

Figure 15.1 7 mm lesion suspicious of a basal cell carcinoma on the left pinna.

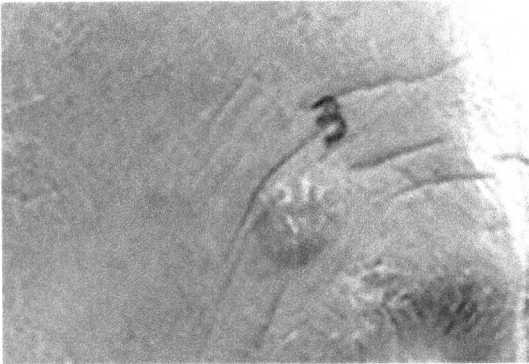

Figure 15.2 Nodular lesion right forehead.

Table 15.2 Glasgow 7-Point Checklist

Major Features	Minor Features
Change in size	Diameter ≥7 mm
Irregular shape	Inflammation
Irregular colour	Oozing
	Change in sensation (including itch)

Table 15.3 Clinical Features of Each Skin Cancer

Cutaneous Malignancy	Clinical Features
Basal cell carcinoma	• Slowly growing plaque or nodule • Prominent telangiectasia around the lesion • Pearly nodule • Skin-coloured, pink or pigmented • Spontaneous bleeding or ulceration
Squamous cell carcinoma	• Grow over weeks to months • Raised, tender nodule • Ulcerated irregular plaques
Cutaneous melanoma	• See Table 15.2 • Initially flat during horizontal growth phase • Raised, nodular following vertical phase • Can lack pigment – amelanotic melanoma

Management

The principles of management in patients with cutaneous malignancy are dependent on the patient's motivation for treatment, medical comorbidities and the underlying pathology. The diagnosis is critical to directing treatment efficiently and effectively and the cornerstones of this include dermoscopic assessment and tissue biopsy.

Clinic investigations

- Bloods – not routinely required in a clinic setting but can be employed for a baseline status
- Dermoscopy (Table 15.4)
- Full-body skin mapping where appropriate in confirmed melanoma patients
- Referral to ophthalmology for slit-lamp biomicroscopy to exclude ocular melanoma in cutaneous melanoma cases
- Biopsy
  - Incisional biopsy – diagnostic uncertainty with a non-pigmented lesion
  - Typically, biopsies are not required for BCC's unless there is uncertainty over the diagnosis, or the lesion is in a critical site on the face such as the nose or medial canthus
  - Pigmented lesions suspected to be melanoma should be excised with a 2 mm clinical margin. If this is not possible due to the size of the lesion, mapping geographic biopsies of key representative areas should be undertaken

Imaging

- USS ± FNAC – cervical lymphadenopathy, parotid masses
- CT – fixed lesions of the scalp
- MRI neck with contrast – clinical cervical lymphadenopathy
- CT chest – completion of staging in SCC to identify distant metastasis
- US FNA, PET-CT and MRI brain only in melanoma greater than stage IIIc

Table 15.4 Dermoscopic Findings Associated with Different Types of Cutaneous Malignancy

Basal Cell Carcinoma	Squamous Cell Carcinoma	Cutaneous Melanoma

• Large blue-grey ovoid nests
• Multiple blue-grey dots and globules
• Leaf-like structures
• Spoke-wheel-like structures
• Arborizing telangiectasia
• Ulceration
• Shiny white blotches and strands
	• Central mass of keratin
	• Targetoid hair follicles
	• Ulceration
		• Menzies criteria
		• Negative features (both must be absent)
		• Symmetry of pigmentation pattern
		• Single colour
		• Positive features (at least one):
		  • Blue-white veil
		  • Multiple brown dots
		  • Pseudopods
		  • Radial streaming
		  • Scar-like depigmentation
		  • Peripheral black dots/globules
		  • Multiple (5–6) colours
		  • Multiple blue-grey dots
		  • Broadened network

Medical

- High-risk BCCs – non-surgical treatments not recommended
- Low-risk BCCs – topical agents (e.g., 5-fluorouracil, imiquimod) or photodynamic therapy (PDT) with topical methyl aminolevulinate (MAL)
- Radiotherapy may be the treatment option if a patient is unable or unwilling to undergo surgery
- cSCC – PDT, radiotherapy, curretage and cautery are non-surgical options generally reserved for patients who decline surgery or are not surgical candidates with low-risk well-defined tumours
- Invasive melanoma – no role for non-surgical treatment

Surgical

BCC

- Excision with a predetermined margin (4–5 mm)

SCC

- Excision margins determined by risk classification
  - 4 mm – low-risk, well-defined tumours (≤20 mm) (excluding the ear and lip)
  - 6 mm – high-risk tumours, 20–40 mm diameter, present on ear or lip or immunocompromised patients
  - 10 mm – very high-risk tumours, >40 mm diameter or solid-organ recipient

Melanoma

- Excision margins determined by the Breslow thickness

- Stage IA (<0.8 mm) – excision with a 1 cm margin
- Stage IB (<0.8 mm with ulceration or 0.8–2 mm) – 1 cm margin and sentinel lymph node biopsy (SLNB)
- Stage II (any tumour thickness without regional metastasis) – 2 cm margin and SLNB
- Stage III or higher – 2 cm margin and appropriate management of the regional metastasis

Discharge and follow-up

BCC

- First BCC – discharged after postoperative review
- Multiple previous BCCs / aggressive histological features / close margin (≤1 mm) – 1-year follow-up
- Genetic syndrome with predisposition to further keratinocyte cancers – lifelong follow-up
- Advise on minimising sun exposure, SPF-50 and a wide-brim hat

cSCC

- Low risk – discharged
- High risk – 2-year follow-up
- Very high risk – 3-year follow-up

Melanoma

- Stage IA – 1-year follow-up
- Others – 3-year follow-up with patient-tailored imaging performed at regular intervals

When to refer from primary care

- Referral via cancer pathway for any suspected melanoma
- Do not biopsy in primary care
- Referral for suspected BCC as routine / urgent but not on cancer pathway unless there is particular concern that a delay may have a significant impact (e.g., due to site or size)

Red flags

- Pigmented lesion meeting either ABCDE or Glasgow criteria
- Rapidly growing lesion
- Ulcerated and bleeding
- Cervical or parotid lymphadenopathy
- Fixity to the underlying tissues

MCQs

1) A 55-year-old fit and well builder attends your secondary care clinic with a 2-month history of an enlarging lesion on the pinna, which occasionally bleeds and is painful. You examine the lesion, and it is 15 mm in diameter, with evidence of ulceration and surrounding skin damage. Which of these would be the most appropriate management?

   A) Excision with 4 mm margin
   B) Excision with 6 mm margin
   C) Curettage and cautery
   D) Radiotherapy
   E) Photodynamic therapy

2) Following excision of the lesion in Question 1, the pathology shows a moderately differentiated cutaneous SCC >1 mm from all margins, no PNI/LVI. How would you follow-up with the patient?

   A) Discharge with advice
   B) 1 years
   C) 2 years
   D) 3 years
   E) 5 years

3) A 78-year-old patient presents with a 3 cm mixed pigmented lesion with an irregular border, at the right temple just lateral to the lateral canthus. She is otherwise fit and well. She is a retired gardener and keen walker. What is the best initial course of management?

   A) Excision with a 1 cm margin and full-thickness skin graft
   B) Excision with a 2 cm margin and split-thickness skin graft
   C) Radiotherapy
   D) Excision with a 2 mm margin
   E) Mapping biopsies

Chapter 16

Salivary gland disease

Keshav K. Gupta and Ahmed Abdelrahman

Background

Salivary gland diseases represent a significant subset of conditions encountered in the realm of maxillofacial surgery, bearing considerable implications for patient quality of life and oral health. These glands, comprising the parotid, submandibular, and sublingual glands, play a pivotal role in the maintenance of oral hygiene, facilitating digestion, and protecting the oral cavity from microbial invasion through the production of saliva. Salivary gland diseases encompass a wide spectrum of disorders that can affect both the quantity and quality of saliva, leading to significant impacts on oral and systemic health. Pathologies affecting the salivary glands can range from inflammatory conditions, such as sialadenitis, to neoplastic processes, including both benign and malignant tumours. This chapter will focus on the surgical management of salivary gland neoplasm and obstructive sialadenopathy.

History

Symptoms

- Onset, timing and duration
- Laterality
- Progression – fluctuating or stable size
- Pain
- Exacerbating or relieving factors (e.g., meals with sialolithiasis)
- Preceding illness (e.g., URTI or other viral illness)
- Associated symptoms – dry mouth, foul taste / purulent discharge, facial pain, facial weakness

Systems

- Airway – difficulty in breathing, SOB, aspiration / choking, drooling
- Oesophagus – dysphagia, odynophagia
- Oral cavity – trismus, oral blood
- Voice – change in voice
- Systemic features / autoimmune – unexplained persistent fever, weight loss, malnutrition, night sweats, reduced appetite, dry eyes, rashes

DOI: 10.1201/9781003493310-18

Table 16.1 Salivary Gland Disease

Infective	Bacterial (*Staphylococcus aureus*), viral (coxsackievirus, parainfluenza, influenza, mumps, HIV, parvovirus B19, herpes), TB
Inflammatory (sialadenitis)	Sjögren's syndrome, granulomatosis with polyangiitis, sarcoidosis
Neoplasm (benign)	Pleomorphic adenoma, Warthin's tumour
Neoplasm (malignant)	Mucoepidermoid carcinoma, adenoid cystic carcinoma, acinic cell carcinoma, ex-pleomorphic adenoma, adenocarcinoma, SCC, lymphoma
Structural	Sialolithiasis (stone), sialectasis (stricture)

Past medical history

- History of autoimmune conditions
- Dental history
- Previous head and neck surgery or radiotherapy
- Use of anticholinergic medication that can reduce salivary production

Social history

- Smoking, alcohol status
- Nutritional status
- Performance status
- Impact on quality of life, activities of daily living and hobbies

Red flags

- Firm, painless mass
- Increasing in size
- Facial nerve weakness
- Paraesthesia/anaesthesia of overlying skin
- Overlying skin changes
- Lump fixation
- Trismus

Examination

- General inspection – asymmetry/swelling, visible masses, skin changes (erythema/ulceration)
- Complete head and neck examination including scalp for skin lesions (cutaneous SCC metastasising to intraparotid lymph nodes)
- Oral cavity
  - Visible stone at duct orifice
  - Mucosal changes – inflammation, discharge, ranulas (mucous retention cysts)

- Assess for xerostomia (moisture level of oral mucosa and tongue)
  - Palpate deep parotid lobe (bimanual palpation from zygomatic arch down to angle of mandible) – size, consistency, tenderness
  - Transillumination – differentiate cystic and hard masses
  - Dentition
- Inspect gland orifices
  - Submandibular and sublingual (Wharton's duct) – floor of the mouth either side of lingual frenulum
  - Parotid (Stensen's duct) – buccal surface by second upper molar (parotid)
- Salivary gland mass
  - Size (parotid swellings can be anteroinferior to the ear lobe), site, overlying skin changes, mobility, pain
- Duct function assessment
  - Milking the gland – assess quantity, quality (clear, mucoid, purulent), ease of flow
  - Taste test – subjective assessment of taste
- Neck – range of motion, palpation for lymphadenopathy
- Voice – quality, volume, hoarseness, pitch
- Signs of respiratory distress and stridor
- Cranial nerves (especially VII)
- TMJ – TMJ disorders may mimic or contribute to salivary gland pathology

Management

The principle of management for patients with salivary gland masses is to distinguish between neoplastic and non-neoplastic causes. Obstructive sialadenopathy is primarily caused by the blockage of salivary flow due to the presence of salivary stones (sialolithiasis), ductal strictures or external compression. The management of this condition depends on the severity of the obstruction, the symptoms and the underlying cause. The goals of treatment are to relieve the obstruction, restore normal salivary flow, and prevent complications such as infection or chronic gland dysfunction. The management of salivary gland neoplasms depends on several factors, including the histological type, size, location, grade and stage of the tumour, as well as the patient's overall health. The primary goal of treatment is to achieve complete tumour resection while preserving function and minimising morbidity often with MDT input.

Bedside tests

- Swab – purulent intraoral discharge (mc&s)
- Bloods
  - FBC, U&Es, CRP, blood cultures – if suspecting infection / abscess
  - Autoimmune screen, HIV test

Imaging

- US ± FNAC
  - Best first-line investigation of solid masses
  - Cytology – benign or malignant
  - Can help exclude abscess in acute setting

- MRI (in neoplasm)
  - Detailed assessment of extent of lesion
  - Relationship of mass to local anatomical structures (e.g., facial nerve)
  - Preoperative planning
- CT neck and chest
  - Staging in confirmed malignancy

Treatment options

Sialadenitis (gland inflammation secondary to infection or autoimmune disease)

- A to E approach because patients may present with airway complications or neck abscess
- Conservative – warm compress, analgesia, hydration, oral hygiene advice
- Medical – antibiotics (oral or IV), analgesia (NSAIDs)
- Rheumatology input if autoimmune cause
- Surgical – parotid abscess can be drained under US guidance

Sialolithiasis (salivary gland stone – more common in submandibular gland)

- Conservative – massage and sialogogues (citrus sweets/fluids that stimulate saliva production)
- Medical – antibiotics (acute infective flare-up), analgesia (NSAIDs)
- Surgery
  - Intraoral ductal stone – ductal excision and extraction
  - Sialendoscopy – for small stones <4 mm
  - Lithotripsy (ESWL) – fragment larger stones to be expelled naturally or removed endoscopically
  - Submandibular gland excision – larger stones intraglandular or at hilum, recurrent disease (Figure 16.1)
  - Ranula – marsupialisation or complete excision

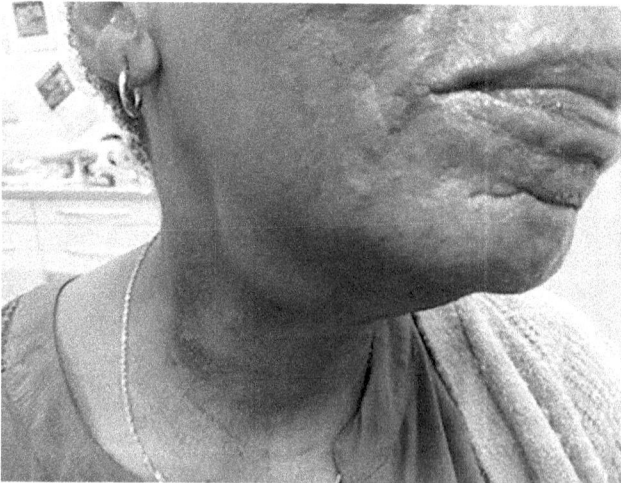

Figure 16.1 Right submandibular salivary gland swelling secondary to stone obstruction.

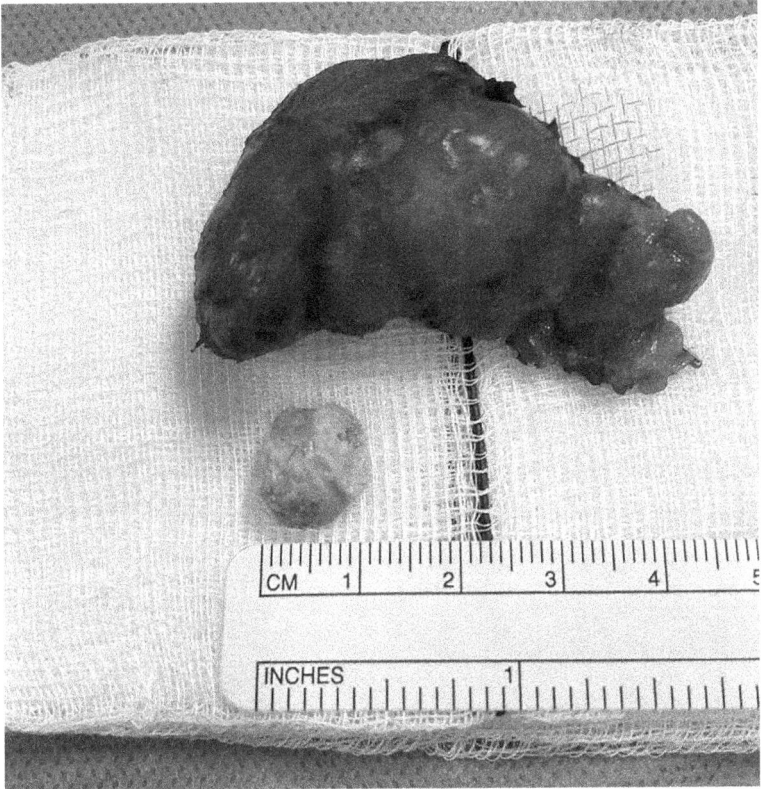

Figure 16.2 Submandibular gland excision with sialolithiasis following surgical excision.

Neoplasm

- Benign
  - Superficial parotidectomy (if deep lobe not involved)
  - Submandibular or sublingual gland excision
  - Enucleation or conservative excision – small well-circumscribed tumours of minor salivary glands
- Malignant
  - Head and neck MDT
  - Surgical – superficial or total parotidectomy (facial nerve sacrificed if involved) or submandibular gland excision ± neck dissection (regional LN metastases)
  - Radiotherapy
    - Primary – inoperable tumours for palliation
    - Postoperative (adjuvant) – high-risk tumours (e.g., >4 cm, residual neck disease, adenoid cystic carcinoma)
  - Reconstruction – to restore function and aesthetics in cases of significant tissue resection

- Adjuvant therapy – radiotherapy or chemotherapy
- Recurrent or metastatic disease – consider revision surgery, radiotherapy, or palliation

Indications for adjuvant therapy

- High-grade malignancies
- Positive surgical margins
- Perineural invasion
- Advanced locoregional disease
- Advanced metastatic disease

Discharge and follow-up

- Follow-up is dependent on the underlying diagnosis and patient factors
- Most cases require long-term follow-up with active surveillance to assess for recurrence that can be even 10–15 years later

MCQs

1) Which of the following is the most common cause of obstructive sialadenopathy?

A) Ductal stricture
B) Sialolithiasis
C) Ranula formation
D) External compression from a mass
E) Autoimmune disease

2) Which of the following is an indication for adjuvant radiotherapy in salivary gland neoplasms?

A) Small, well-circumscribed benign tumours
B) Tumour more than 4 cm in size
C) Tumours confined to the superficial parotid lobe
D) Acute sialadenitis with abscess formation
E) Intraoral ductal stones

3) Which management strategy is most appropriate for a symptomatic salivary stone less than 4 mm in size?

A) Submandibular gland excision
B) Sialendoscopy
C) Lithotripsy
D) Ductal excision and extraction
E) Conservative management with massage and sialogogues

Chapter 17

Head and neck reconstruction (free flaps)

Farhan Khalid and Sat Parmar

Background

Free flaps are either soft tissue (skin, subcutaneous tissue, fascia, muscle) or composite (with bone) harvested from a distant part of the body with its own blood supply (pedicle) and anastomosed to neck vessels close to the surgical defect. They are considered to be the gold standard for head and neck reconstruction on the reconstruction ladder due to their pliability, precision, variation in size and shape and ability to maintain movement of the head and neck. They aim to replace like for like. In addition, they have advantages of restoring form and function with better outcomes for patients compared to regional pedicled flaps which are based on axial blood supply close to head and neck area (for example a pectoralis major myocutaneous flap).

In OMFS, free flaps are generally used in cases of head and neck cancer, especially of the oral cavity. Surgical resection of oral cavity tumours often involves extensive soft tissue or hard tissue resection. This can lead to devastating functional (speech, swallow, mastication, oral competence) and cosmetic deficits which can in turn compromise a patient's nutritional, physical and psychological health and thus their quality of life. In addition to ablative surgery for head and neck malignancy, head and neck free flap reconstruction can also be utilised in the management of trauma, congenital deformities, infections and benign conditions and in cases of osteoradionecrosis of the jaw.

This chapter will focus on how to clinically assess patients for suitability for head and neck free flap reconstruction.

History

Tissue factors

- Assess for vessel quality – intermittent claudication, radiotherapy to the neck
- Assess for tissue quality – donor site scars, radiotherapy to the neck

Patient factors

- Comorbidities – especially heart failure, IHD, PVD, COPD, dementia, coagulopathies, DVT
- Smoking

DOI: 10.1201/9781003493310-19

Examination

- General inspection
- Tumour assessment
  - Size, site, extent, accessibility
- Donor site assessment
  - Previous surgery, scars, patient preference
- Radial forearm free flaps
  - Allen's test (assessment of collateral circulation of hand by compressing arterial inflow of radial and ulnar artery and allowing only ulnar perfusion to assess capillary refill of thumb and index finger)
- Anterolateral thigh flap
  - Handheld Doppler ultrasound of skin to assess perfusion and delineate arterial perforator vessels

Investigations

- OPG – assess dentition
- CT/MRI head and neck – tumour assessment, extent, resectability, assessment of neck vessels (CT gives the advantage of 3D virtual planning and reconstruction)
- CT neck and thorax – staging
- CT/MR angiogram of lower limbs – assessment of collateral blood supply to lower limb if fibula free flap planned

Management

The principles of management in patients using a head and neck free flap is to ensure you are choosing the correct flap for the correct patient for the correct indication. This requires detailed assessment and meticulous planning with involvement of the MDT. Management requires consideration of patient factors (age, sex, body habitus, functional status, general medical and psychological health, available donor sites, previous head and neck cancer treatments, availability of neck vessels for anastomosis and patient's choice), tumour factors (site, size, extent, involved structures, soft tissue or composite [bone and soft tissue] resection and likely need for postoperative radiotherapy) as well as availability of surgical expertise and appropriate resources. Patients also require airway assessments for surgical planning and in order to manage the airway postoperatively often requiring tracheostomy at the time of ablative surgery.

Table 17.1 Flap Selection

Type	Tissue	Blood Supply	Advantages	Disadvantages
Radial forearm free flap (Figure 17.1)	Skin, fascia	Radial artery	Thin, pliable skin paddle, large long pedicle, two teams operating, reliable	Donor site not hidden, need skin grafting and potential for graft loss and tendon exposure, sensory disturbance of forearm
Radial composite flap	Skin, bone	Radial artery	Same as radial forearm free flap but with the advantage of bone for periorbital and perinasal defects	Same as radial forearm free flap and risk of radius fracture
Anterolateral thigh (ALT) flap	Skin, fascia, muscle	Lateral circumflex femoral artery (descending branch)	Skin, fascia, muscle, up to 8 x 25 cm skin paddle, long pedicle, minimal donor site morbidity, two teams operating	Sensory disturbance to lateral thigh, occasional excessive volume of tissue
Rectus abdominis free flap	Muscle, skin, fascia	Deep inferior epigastric artery	Versatile, large area of skin and muscle, reliable, two teams operating	Ileus, hernia, scar, abdominal weakness
Free fibula flap (Figure 17.2)	Skin, fascia, muscle, bone	Peroneal artery	Gold standard for mandibular reconstruction, up to 26 cm of bone can be harvested, long pedicle, two teams operating,	Sensory disturbance of leg, ankle stiffness/ mild instability, graft failure, motor weakness
Iliac crest free flap (DCIA)	Bone, muscle, skin	Deep circumflex iliac artery	Two teams operating, large quantity and height of bone, reliable vessels	Relatively short pedicle, risk of ileus, hernia, chronic pain, femoral paraesthesia
Scapula free flap	Skin, fascia, muscle, bone	Circumflex scapular artery	Versatile, option of using bone, multiple skin paddles, muscle for large complex reconstruction, adequate pedicle length, reliable vessels	Stiffness and limitation of shoulder movements, scar, single team operating, longer anaesthetic time

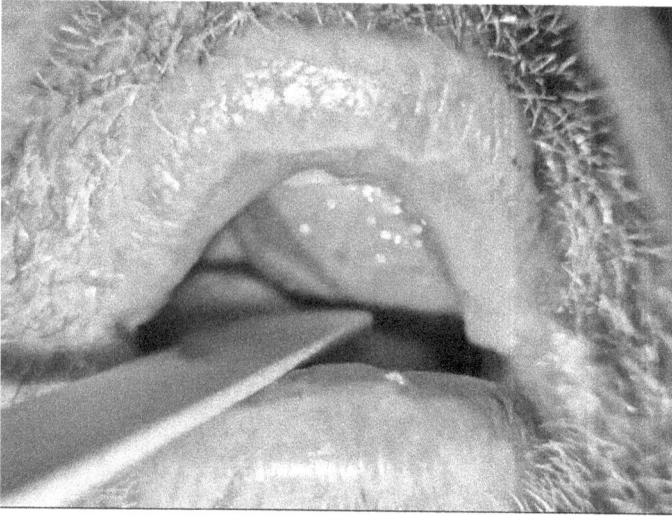

Figure 17.1 Intraoral image of a radial forearm free flap used to reconstruct a soft palate defect following SCC resection.

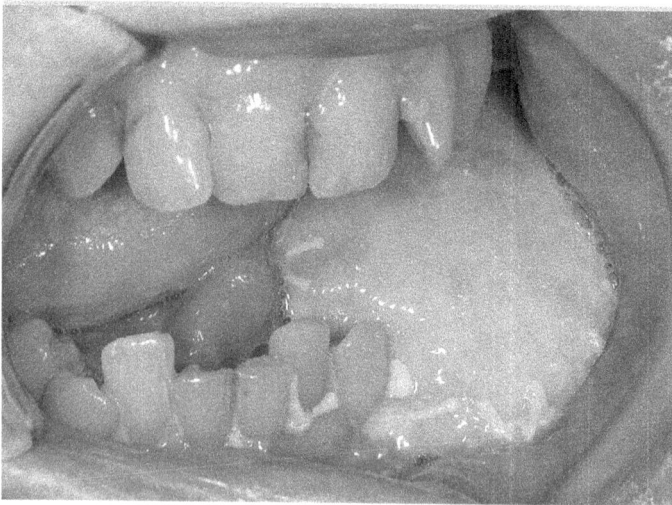

Figure 17.2 Intraoral left soft tissue skin paddle from fibula free flap reconstruction for oral cavity SCC.

MCQs

1) The most widely used free flap for mandibular reconstruction is

   A) Scapula free flap
   B) Iliac crest free flap
   C) Radial forearm free flap
   D) Fibula free flap
   E) Iliac crest flap

2) The main disadvantage of using free flaps for head and neck reconstructions is

   A) Suboptimal functional
   B) Donor site morbidity
   C) Poor cosmesis
   D) Contraction
   E) Scarring

3) The main advantage of free flap reconstruction is

   A) Better functional and cosmetic outcomes
   B) Equivocal outcomes
   C) Variation of treatment options
   D) 100% success rate
   E) Patient choice

Orthognathic surgery

Ashwin Kerai

Background

Orthognathic surgery is performed to correct dentofacial disproportion (facial deformity or facial asymmetry) and requires an MDT approach to plan treatment, typically involving orthodontists, psychologists and dental technicians in addition to the OMFS surgeons. Preoperative planning with a thorough history, examination and appropriate investigations is vital to ensure a successful outcome. Orthognathic surgery is typically performed electively and as such it is vital to establish the patient's concerns and motivation for treatment in order to achieve a final result that both the clinician and patient are happy with. In terms of facial asymmetry, all patients will have this to some degree. However, it is important to identify cases in which significant facial asymmetry is the underlying cause and potential management options differ from the approach in routine orthognathic surgery. There are a number of possible causes of facial asymmetry, and a thorough history, systematic examination and special investigations are the cornerstone to identifying the cause and providing the correct treatment plan.

History

Symptoms – may be variable and include functional and aesthetic concerns

- Onset, timing and duration
- Better or worse
- Triggers
- Preceding trauma

Systems

- Aesthetic – dental/facial appearance, screening for body dysmorphic disorder
- Dental – difficulty biting or chewing (e.g., anterior open bite or significant reverse overjet), malocclusion, TMJ dysfunction, appearance
- Throat – sleep apnoea
- Voice – change in voice/speech difficulties

Past medical history

- Craniofacial syndromes
- Inflammatory arthropathies (can contribute to class II) or acromegaly (class III)

DOI: 10.1201/9781003493310-20

- States of immunocompromise
- Coagulopathies
- Previous surgery or radiotherapy
- Medications – bisphosphonates, anticoagulants, steroids, oral contraception

Red flags/Risk factors

- Body dysmorphic disorder
- Progressive mandibular asymmetry
  - Unilateral condylar hyperplasia
  - Unilateral condylar resorption
  - Condylar tumour e.g., osteochondroma
  - Hemi-mandibular elongation
  - Hemi-mandibular hypertrophy
- Acromegaly
  - Progressive post-pubertal mandibular growth
  - Associated craniofacial signs and symptoms such as frontal bossing, macro-glossia, interdental spacing, class III skeletal and incisal relationship
- Idiopathic condylar resorption
  - Gradual increase in anterior open bite
  - Can be triggered by orthodontic treatment or orthognathic surgery
  - High-angle class II skeletal pattern

Red flags for body dysmorphic disorder

- Patient's concerns appear out of proportion to the extent of deformity
- Preoccupation and excessive and intrusive thoughts regarding the perceived deformity triggering anxiety, depression and distress
- Lack of insight that the perceived deformity is absent or minimal
- Impairment of function and attributing concerns to life events such as relationship breakdowns or unemployment
- Avoids social contact
- May have sought numerous options and have had previous objectively good results but still be dissatisfied

Social history

- Jehovah's Witness – maxilla surgery has the potential for high blood loss
- Smoking – wound healing and periodontal disease
- Hobbies – no contact sports 6 weeks post-surgery, wind and brass instruments require full sensation to the lower lip

Examination

- General points – consider ethnicity and racial norms, examine in a natural head posture with the patient relaxed (facial soft tissue in resting positions)
- General inspection of the face – features of a craniofacial syndrome
- General inspection of stature and body form
- Assess BMI – both BMI extremes can have deleterious effects during and following surgery

- Systemic – hands (acromegaly), limbs (craniofacial syndromes)
- Frontal facial examination
  - Facial asymmetry
  - Cranial base – look at position of ears and check for orbital dystopia
  - Orbits – symmetry, dystopia, intercanthal distance
  - Nose – nasal dorsum width two-thirds of intercanthal distance; alar base should equal intercanthal distance
  - Nasolabial angle – 100° (± 10°) greater in females than males
  - Upper lip length – subnasale to upper lip stomion
    - Male – 22 ± 2 mm
    - Female – 20 ± 2 mm
  - Incisor show – upper incisor show should be 2.5 mm (± 1.5 mm) in repose; 1–2 mm of gingival exposure on smiling
  - Midlines – facial midline, chin midline, dental midline should all be coincident to each other
  - Chin throat angle 110°
  - Soft tissues – infraorbital, paranasal hollowing
- Lateral facial examination
  - Position of the maxilla relative to line of zero meridian (vertical line downwards from nasion and perpendicular to the Frankfort horizontal plane)
  - Skeletal pattern – chin projection assessed relative to maxilla position
    - Class I – chin point in line with maxilla
    - Class II – chin point behind
    - Class III – chin point ahead

Differential diagnosis

Dentofacial deformities

- Class II skeletal pattern
  - with vertical maxillary excess
  - with vertical maxillary deficiency
- Class III skeletal pattern
  - with vertical maxillary excess
- Any combination of these with mandibular asymmetry

Facial asymmetry

- Congenital – craniosynostosis, cleft, microsomia, linea scleroderma, syndromes (Parry – Romberg, Treacher Collins)
- Acquired (categorised according to mandibular growth)
  - Normal – deformational plagiocephaly, torticollis, condylar dislocation, mandibular posturing
  - Restricted – TMJ ankylosis, radiotherapy, condylar resorption, inflammatory arthropathies
  - Increased – benign (osteochondroma, osteoma), pre-malignant (synovial chondromatosis), malignant (osteosarcoma)

Management

The principles of management with dentofacial deformities are combined orthodontic and orthognathic surgery. All patients should be seen and assessed within a joint orthognathic clinic with an orthognathic surgeon and orthodontist present. A full evaluation as described tailoring the patient's concerns to the objective findings of the assessment provides the basis of the majority of management plans.

Imaging – holistic imaging helps to evaluate the patient's face, dental occlusion and help with surgical planning

- Photographs
    - Standard facial views at rest and smiling; lateral and lateral oblique views at rest and smiling
    - Intraoral views – upper and lower dental arch; teeth in occlusion
- Study models
    - Surgical planning requires cast models mounted on an adjustable articular
- Radiographs
    - OPG – pathology, condylar pathology and wisdom teeth
    - Lateral cephalogram – cephalometric analysis, orthodontic planning
    - Posteroanterior cephalogram / CT scan – cases of asymmetry
- SPECT-CT 99mTC radionucleotide scan – highlights osteoblastic activity

Non-operative (orthodontic)

- Mild skeletal deformities
- Dental aesthetic concerns are the forefront to the patient
- Unfit for surgery
- Patient wishes

Surgical

- Can be performed any time after growth cessation
- Pre-surgical (orthodontic) phase
    - Fixed appliances
    - Relieve dental crowding, level and align the arches, decompensate, coordinate the arches
- Maxillary surgery
    - Osteotomies based on Le Fort fracture lines
    - Most commonly Le Fort I osteotomy (sulcus incision)
        - Nasal intubation
        - Medical adjuncts – IV tranexamic acid, dexamethasone, antibiotics
- Mandibular surgery
    - Commonly bilateral sagittal split osteotomy – to advance / setback / correct asymmetry

- Genioplasty
  - Standalone or adjunct procedure – allow chin position to be moved/
    changed
    - AP plane – advanced
    - Vertical dimension – augmented or reduced
    - Rotated left/right to correct midline discrepancy
    - Transverse dimension – widened or narrowed
- Condylectomy – standalone or adjunct procedure
- TMJ replacement

Other surgical techniques

- High Le Fort I osteotomy
- Le Fort II osteotomy
- Le Fort III osteotomy
- Segmental maxillary surgery
- Inverted L osteotomy of mandible
- Vertical sagittal split osteotomy of the mandible
- Segmental mandibular osteotomies
  - Kole osteotomy
  - Total subapical osteotomy

Discharge and follow-up

- Patients will typically spend one to two nights in hospital postoperatively
- Soft diet 6 weeks
- Avoid contact sports
- Excellent oral hygiene
- Follow-up usually 6 months postoperatively to finalise dental occlusion and
  photographs as reference
- Lifelong retention (usually removable retainers worn at night)

Complications of orthognathic surgery

- Bleeding – pterygoid venous plexus, greater palatine pedicle, nasopalatine ves-
  sels or maxillary artery
- Unfavourable osteotomy of the mandible
- Nerve damage – inferior alveolar
- Condylar positioning
- Tooth damage
- Non-union
- Relapse and poor stability

MCQs

1) A 23-year-old patient is undergoing a Le Fort I osteotomy. During the down-fracture the surgeon experiences significant bleeding. The first most appropriate management is to

A) Transfuse packed red cells
B) Ligate the external carotid artery
C) Transfer the patient to angiography for embolisation
D) Ask the anaesthetist to reduce the blood pressure further
E) Pack the maxilla and apply upward pressure

2) A 35-year-old male patient attends your clinic unhappy with the appearance of his chin because he feels it is set back too far. His past medical history includes anxiety. He has a large dorsal hump. He has previously sought an opinion from a plastic surgeon for a chin implant. He feels his weak chin is impacting his ability to gain promotion at work. What is an appropriate management strategy for this patient?

A) Suggest referral directly to a psychologist
B) Suggest a rhinoplasty may provide facial harmony
C) Refer the patient to a colleague for assessment
D) Refuse to treat the patient because you do not feel his concerns are valid
E) Review the patient in an orthognathic MDT with a psychologist

3) You are performing bimaxillary surgery in which there is a significant impaction of the maxilla followed by advancement of the mandible. There were some difficulties in positioning the maxilla initially. After carrying out the mandibular surgery, the intermaxillary fixation is released and it is noted that there is an anterior open bite when the final wafer is removed, and the occlusion checked. The most likely cause of this is

A) Relapse of the mandible
B) An unfavourable split on one side of the mandible
C) Fixation failure of the osteosynthesis plate
D) Incorrect condylar positioning
E) Insufficient release of the soft tissue envelope

Chapter 19

TMJ disorders

Daanesh Zakai and Clayton Davis

Background

The temporomandibular joint (TMJ) is one of the most complex joints in the human body, facilitating crucial functions such as chewing, speaking and other facial movements. It connects the mandible to the temporal bone of the skull and operates via both rotational and translational movements (ginglymoarthrodial joint). Dysfunction in the TMJ can result in temporomandibular joint disorders (TMDs), which are characterised by pain, restricted movement and functional impairment. TMDs can arise from various causes including trauma, degenerative diseases (e.g., osteoarthritis or rheumatoid arthritis), congenital deformities and tumours affecting the TMJ.

History

Symptoms

- Onset, timing and duration
- Laterality
- Triggers or alleviating factors – e.g., chewing, talking
- Preceding factors – e.g., surgery, trauma, jaw dislocation

Systems

- Dental – dental decay/infections due to inability to maintain oral care
- Ear – tinnitus, otalgia, ear infections
- Orthopaedic – recurrent swelling in other joints
- Voice – difficulty in speech due to progressive limitation in opening

Risk factors/Red flags

- Severe pain despite treatment
- Neurological symptoms – numbness, tingling, weakness
- Systemic symptoms – fever, weight loss, fatigue
- Unexplained jaw deformity
- Persistent jaw locking

DOI: 10.1201/9781003493310-21

Past medical history

- Previous episodes
- Previous TMJ surgery/dental procedures

Examination

- General inspection – body habitus, facial asymmetry, incisal opening, lateral excursive and protrusive movements of jaw
- Joints – palpation of joints for clicking, crepitus, dislocation, locking
- Oral cavity – tongue or floor-of-mouth swelling, dental infections, trismus, occlusion
- Neck – range of motion, cervical lymphadenopathy

Management

The principles of management of TMJ disorders are to aim to restore normal joint function as best as possible. Management can be in a stepwise approach ranging from conservative options such as medications and physiotherapy to TJR. The gold standard for replacement of the TMJ is the custom prosthesis which can take up to 3 months to design and produce (Figure 19.1).

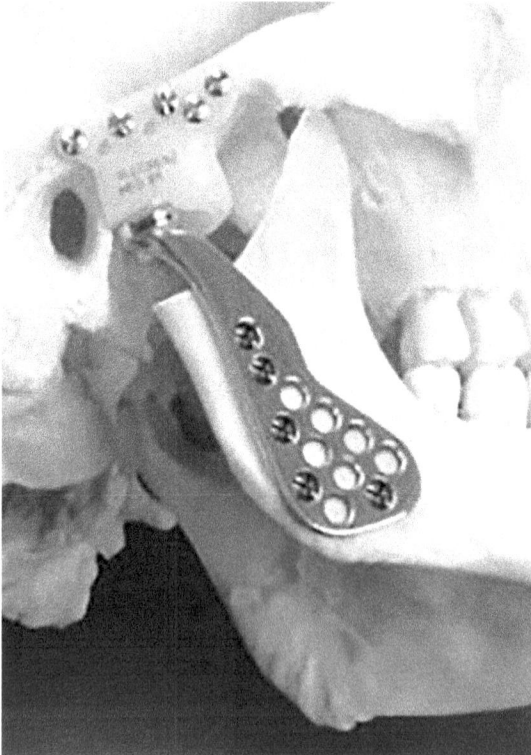

Figure 19.1 Custom right TMJ replacement prosthesis.

Bedside

- Bloods – not usually indicated, can be performed as a baseline

Imaging

- CT – evaluate extent of joint degeneration or ankylosis
- MRI – assessing articular disc and joint capsule

Conservative

- Dental bite guards
- Physiotherapy
- Analgesia (NSAIDs)
- Muscle relaxants

Surgical (TMJ replacement)

- Involvement of the MDT
- Custom prosthesis to replace the diseased joint (can be stock devices)

Discharge and follow-up

- Patients can be discharged once pain is controlled
- Postoperative radiographs may be indicated to check alignment (Figure 19.2)
- Diet – soft diet recommended
- Activity restrictions – avoid strenuous activity that may impact the jaw
- Follow-up – every 4–6 weeks to monitor prosthetic function
- Community nursing teams – if dressing or wound care input is needed

When to refer from primary care

To ED

- Severe, unrelenting pain
- Neurological symptoms or systemic signs
- Rapidly worsening jaw deformity
- Inability to open or close the mouth

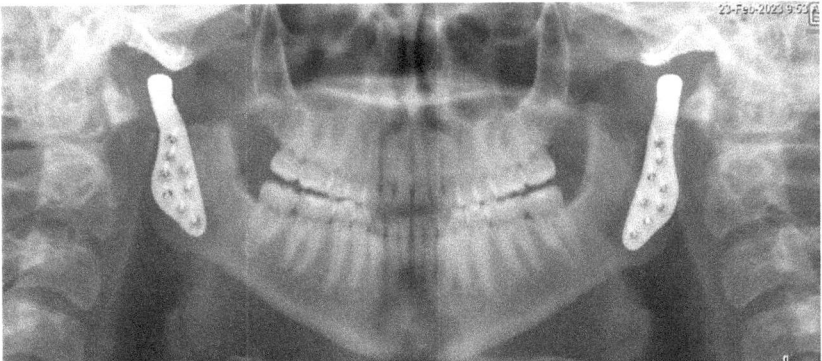

Figure 19.2 Postoperative XR of a bilateral TMJR.

To trauma clinic

- Jaw injuries associated with significant trauma
- Complex cases needing specialist surgical intervention

To clinic via cancer referral pathway

- Suspicious lesions in the TMJ area
- Persistent, unexplained symptoms suggesting malignancy

To routine clinic

- Chronic TMJ symptoms not responding to primary care interventions
- Need for long-term management and follow-up

MCQs

1) Which of the following is NOT a common indication for TMJ replacement?

   A) Rheumatoid arthritis
   B) Severe trauma to the mandible
   C) Temporalis muscle hyperplasia
   D) Ankylosis of the joint
   E) Osteoarthritis

2) Which imaging modality is best for evaluating soft tissues of TMJ?

   A) X-ray
   B) Ultrasound
   C) MRI
   D) CT scan
   E) PET scan

3) To which alloy component in the TMJR are patients commonly allergic?

   A) Titanium
   B) Molybdenum
   C) Nickel
   D) Cobalt
   E) Silver

Chapter 20

TMJ ankylosis

Daanesh Zakai and Clayton Davis

Background

Temporomandibular joint (TMJ) ankylosis refers to the fusion of the mandibular condyle to the temporal bone, leading to a limitation in the movement of the jaw. This condition can significantly impair basic functions such as chewing, speaking, and in severe cases, breathing. TMJ ankylosis can be classified as either intra-articular (true) or extra-articular (false) based on whether the fusion occurs within the joint itself or outside it. Common causes of TMJ ankylosis include trauma, infection, or systemic diseases such as ankylosing spondylitis or rheumatoid arthritis. The condition can also develop as a complication of surgical procedures in the TMJ area. Patients with TMJ ankylosis often experience progressive difficulty opening their mouths (trismus), leading to nutritional deficiencies, speech impairments and compromised oral hygiene.

Preparation and equipment

TMJ ankylosis can rarely present as an emergency in cases in which airway compromise or severe functional limitations arise. If there is any suspicion of airway obstruction or difficulty in breathing or swallowing, this condition should be treated as an OMFS emergency, and the patient should be seen urgently.

History

Symptoms

- Onset, timing, and duration
- Laterality
- Better or worse – chewing, talking
- Preceding factors – trauma, surgery, infection
- Previous episodes

Systems

- Dental – dental decay/infections due to inability to maintain oral care
- Ear – otalgia, infection, tinnitus
- Joints – swelling in other joints
- Voice – difficulty in speech due to progressive limitation in opening
- Systemic – fever, rash, general malaise

DOI: 10.1201/9781003493310-22

Risk factors/Red flags

- Trauma to the jaw
- Infection (especially ear infections that spread to the TMJ)
- Autoimmune diseases such as rheumatoid arthritis
- Facial asymmetry in children (indicative of developmental issues)

Past medical history

- Previous TMJ surgery (e.g., meniscectomy, ORIF condyle)
- Autoimmune disease
- Genetic conditions with craniofacial abnormalities

Examination

- General inspection – signs of respiratory distress: noisy breathing (stridor or stertor), tachypnoea, cyanosis, use of accessory muscles, fatigue
- Voice – speaking in full sentences, changes in voice quality
- Oral cavity – trismus, tongue or floor-of-the-mouth swelling, dental infections, measure MIO
- Neck – range of motion, lumps, torticollis

Red flags

- Airway obstruction
- Severe trismus
- Facial asymmetry in paediatric patients

Management

The principle of managing TMJ ankylosis requires a well-structured MDT approach, combining surgical and non-surgical options based on severity. Early diagnosis and timely intervention are essential to prevent further complications, especially in paediatric patients in whom ankylosis can result in facial asymmetry and growth disturbances. Treatment typically involves surgical release of the ankylosis and, in some cases, joint reconstruction as a single-stage or two-stage procedure.

MDT members involved in TMJ ankylosis

- Oral and maxillofacial surgeon (lead)
- Anaesthetist (for airway management)
- Radiologist (for imaging and diagnosis)
- Physiotherapist (for postoperative rehabilitation)
- Speech and language therapist (for postoperative speech evaluation)
- Nursing staff (postoperative care)
- Pain management specialist

Bedside

- Bloods – if suspected infection
- Swabs – mc&s from oral cavity or surrounding tissue – if suspected infection/abscess

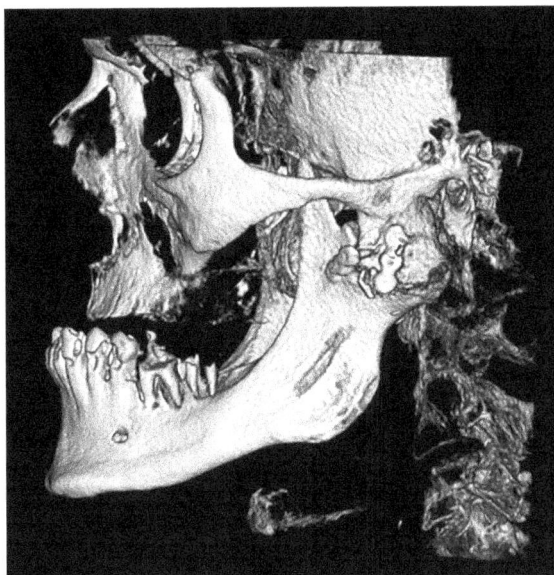

Figure 20.1 TMJ ankylosis secondary to trauma.

Imaging

- CT TMJ – assess extent of bony fusion and ankylosis (Figure 20.1)
- CT angiogram – identify any vessels entering the ankylotic mass which may require embolization prior to surgery (Figure 20.2)
- MRI – assess soft tissue involvement and any inflammatory changes or disc pathology

Conservative

- Physical therapy – physiotherapy and jaw exercises to prevent progression in early disease
- Jaw manipulation – mild cases to restore some movement, often temporary

Medical

- Antibiotics – if infections/abscess

Surgical (Figure 20.3)

- Usually on an elective basis
- Excision of ankylosed joint
- Reconstruction – costochondral grafts or custom alloplastic TMJ prosthesis (single- or two-stage procedure)

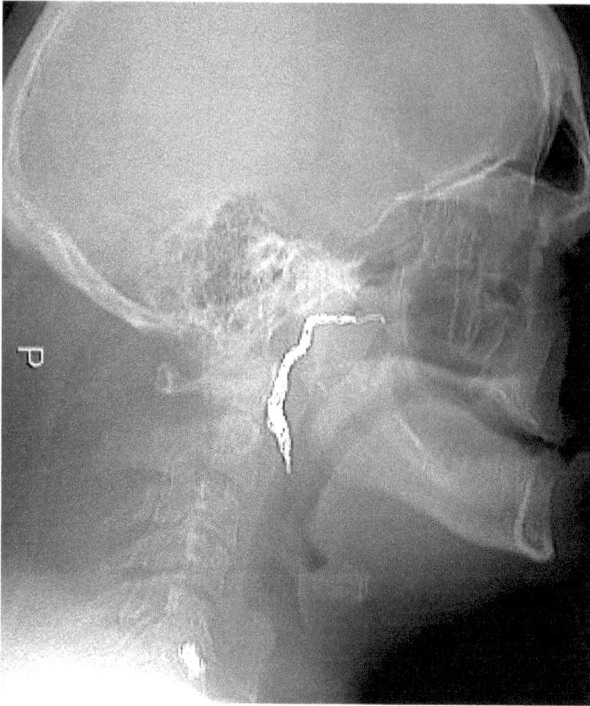

Figure 20.2 CT angiogram with embolization of vessel into the ankylotic mass.

Discharge and follow-up

- Discharge once postoperative pain is controlled and adequate mouth function regained
- Follow-up – every 4–6 weeks to monitor healing and joint function
- Longer follow-up – paediatrics to monitor facial growth and jaw development
- Advice regarding jaw exercises or splints

When to refer from primary care

To ED

- Severe airway compromise or inability to open the mouth

To trauma clinic

- Following facial or mandibular trauma

To routine clinic

- Chronic or progressive TMJ dysfunction without airway issues

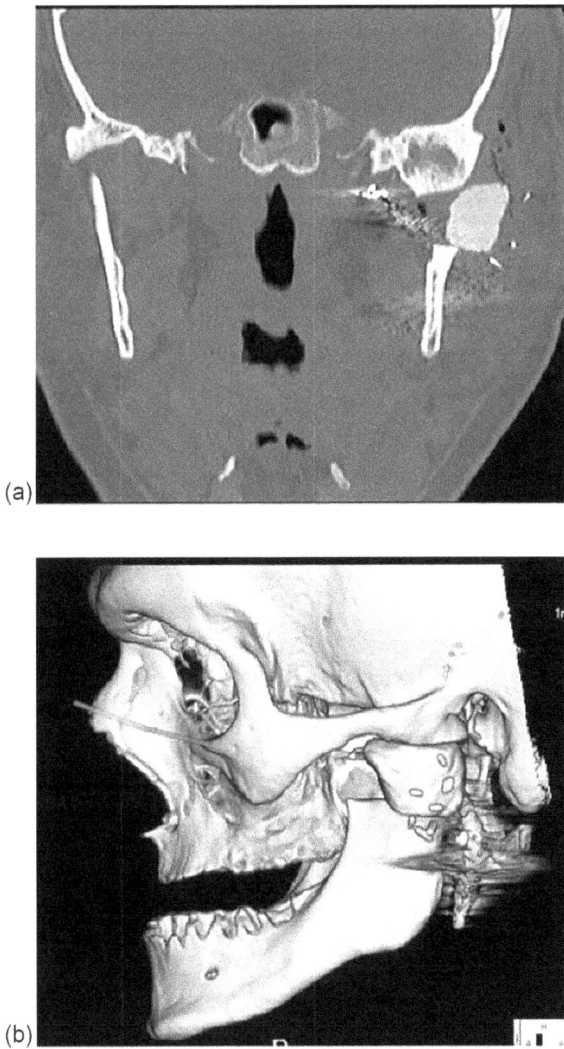

Figure 20.3 First-stage resection of ankylosis (a) and insertion of spacer for subsequent TJR (b).

MCQs

1) Which of the following is a common cause of TMJ ankylosis?

   A) Facial nerve palsy
   B) Viral infection
   C) Trauma to the mandible
   D) Temporalis muscle spasm
   E) Dental abscess

2) Which imaging modality is most useful for assessing bony ankylosis of the TMJ?

   A) X-ray
   B) Ultrasound
   C) MRI
   D) CT scan
   E) PET scan

3) What is the definitive surgical treatment for TMJ ankylosis?

   A) Arthroscopy
   B) Gap arthroplasty with TMJ replacement
   C) Intra articular steroid injection
   D) Joint debridement
   E) Mandibular reconstruction

Chapter 21

Cleft lip and palate

Keshav K. Gupta, Ahmed Abdelrahman and William Breakey

Background

Cleft lip and/or palate is the most prevalent craniofacial anomaly, occurring in approximately 1 in 750 live births in the United Kingdom. The spectrum of this condition ranges from a minor notch in the lip (microform cleft) to a complete bilateral cleft involving both the lip and palate. Cleft lip and palate occur due to a failure in the fusion of embryological facial processes during development. The condition is considered multifactorial, with genetic predisposition pivotal in increasing susceptibility. Environmental factors, such as exposure to teratogenic drugs, nutritional deficiencies, chemicals, radiation and physical obstructions, can also contribute. Cleft lip and palate usually manifest as an isolated anomaly but can occur as part of a syndrome or sequence. Associated syndromes include Stickler's syndrome, Van der Woude syndrome and DiGeorge syndrome, among others.

Depending on its severity, cleft lip and palate can profoundly impact the affected child, their parents, and the healthcare system. These patients require comprehensive and multidisciplinary care over an extended period, highlighting the complexity and significance of managing this condition. There are several classification systems to describe cleft lip and palate deformities based on the embryology and clinical presentation. These provide a way of grouping patients together to aid the management and quantify outcomes. The LAHSHAL system is widely used in the UK and classifies patients according to the extent and severity of their cleft deformity. It describes a cleft from the patient's right side and denotes whether the lip, alveolus, hard palate, or soft palate are affected. A complete cleft is represented by a capital letter. For example, a complete right-sided CLP is denoted as LAHS; a complete left-sided CLP is denoted as SHAL.

Members of the cleft MDT

- Cleft surgeon (OMFS, plastics, or ENT)
- ENT surgeon
- Maxillofacial surgeon
- Specialist cleft nurse
- Paediatric dentist
- Orthodontist
- Speech and language therapist

DOI: 10.1201/9781003493310-23

- Audiologist
- Clinical psychologist
- Clinical geneticist
- Restorative dentist
- Medical photographer

History

Approximately 81% of cleft lip cases are diagnosed antenatally at the 20-week anomaly scan; 60% of patients with a cleft lip have a co-existing cleft palate. Cleft palate is reliably assessed via ultrasound. A referral to the cleft team is made within 24 hours of diagnosis and a cleft specialist nurse will contact the family within 24 hours of receiving the diagnosis. It is important to establish the effects of cleft on a child through history-taking across five main areas:

1) Airway issues
2) Feeding problems
3) Hearing difficulties
4) Psychological concerns (parent and child)
5) Aesthetic concerns

Systems

- Airway – aspiration/choking, drooling
- Oesophagus – dysphagia, odynophagia
- Systemic – extra-cranial features specifically if part of syndrome

Examination

- Full examination of the head and neck including the oral cavity
- Categorisation of cleft deformity as
  - Lip or palate or both (Figure 21.1)
  - Complete or incomplete
  - Unilateral or bilateral
- Assessment for craniofacial abnormalities as part of a wider spectrum
- Dynamic assessment of feeding
- Newborn Hearing Screening Programme (NHSP)

Management

The principle of management in patients with cleft lip/palate is multifaceted and requires an intricate network of multidisciplinary specialists. Aims include restoring the natural appearance of the lip and nose; supporting proper development of speech, language, and auditory functions; and achieving functional alignment of teeth and effective chewing. Longer-term aims include promoting strong oral health, including healthy teeth and gums; and fostering healthy emotional and social development.

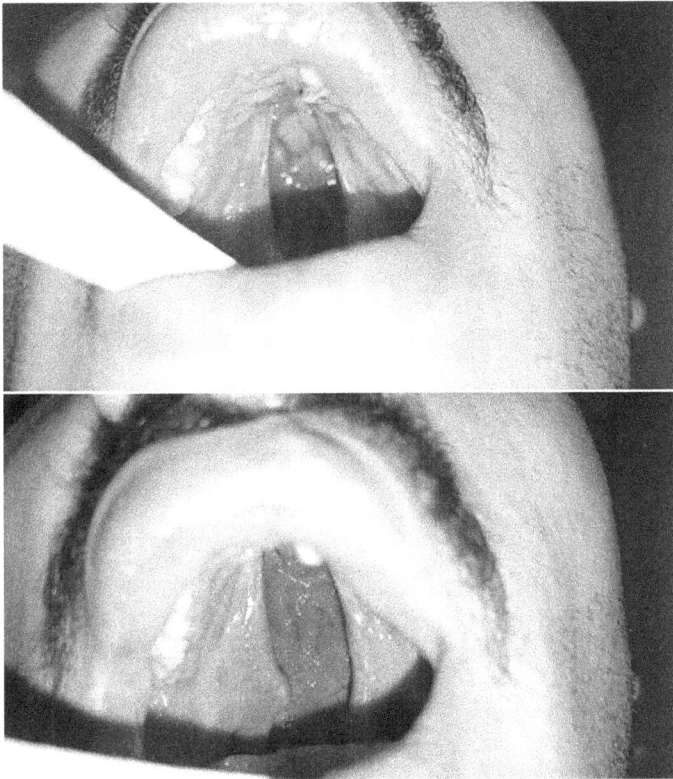

Figure 21.1 Adult patient with a cleft palate (hard and soft palate).

0–3 months

- Cleft nurse input
- Specialist feeding assessment
    - Advice regarding bottle and feed types
    - Aim to avoid NGT where possible
- Clinical psychology support
- NHSP and referral to ENT/audiology as needed

3–6 months (primary palate repair)

- Lip ± hard palate repair surgery
- Lip is repaired by 6 months
    - Layered closure of all tissues and orbicularis oris continuity reinstated – Fisher (anatomical subunit) or Millard (rotation-advancement) repairs
    - Co-existing hard palate repair – vomerine flap closure

6–12 months (secondary palate repair)

- Palate repair surgery
  - Intravelar veloplasty (IVVP or the Sommerlad repair)
  - Layered closure of the nasal mucosa, retropositioning of levator veli palatini, mass closure of the muscle bulk and palate oral layer closure

18 months–5 years

- SLT assessment
  - Aim for good quality intelligible speech at 5 years
- Psychological support
- Paediatric dentistry input
- Audiology and ENT input
  - Hearing rehabilitation
  - Manage glue ear/recurrent infections
- Further surgery if indicated
  - Velopharyngeal insufficiency

6–12 years

- Orthodontic assessment
- Alveolar bone graft (ABG) assessment and surgery after 7 years
  - Bone harvested from the anterior iliac crest

13–20 years

- Genetic counselling/screening
- Orthodontic treatment
- Orthognathic assessment/surgery including osteotomy
  - Jaw repositioning
  - Ameliorate any class 3 malalignment
- Psychological input
- Further surgery if indicated
  - Rhinoplasty
  - Dental surgery
  - Lip revision

MCQs

1) Which of the following is usually carried out in the first 3 months of life in a child with cleft lip/palate?

   A) Lip repair
   B) Palate repair
   C) Hearing test
   D) Alveolar bone graft
   E) Orthodontic assessment

2) Which of the following procedures can be considered in secondary palate repair surgery?

   A) Vomerine flap closure
   B) Fisher repair
   C) Millard repair
   D) Sommerlad repair
   E) Le Fort osteotomy

3) In neonates with a cleft lip and palate, which of the following is usually required?

   A) Nasogastric tube
   B) Specialist feeding bottle
   C) Tracheostomy
   D) Hearing aid
   E) Gastrostomy tube

Chapter 22

Vascular malformation
Ahmed Abdelrahman and Kevin McMillan

Background

Vascular anomalies are broadly categorised into two major groups: tumours and malformations, based on the modified International Society for the Study of Vascular Anomalies (ISSVA) classification. Vascular tumours, such as hemangiomas, fall outside the scope of this chapter. Unlike vascular tumours, vascular malformations are not present at birth and can be divided into low-flow and high-flow lesions. High-flow arteriovenous malformations (AVMs) are locally aggressive lesions which behave clinically as a low-grade neoplasm. They rarely regress and will continue to enlarge with an increased propensity for complications. Accurate diagnosis and staging of the extent of the disease is essential for proper management. Low-flow vascular malformations (venous, capillary, lymphatic, and mixed) are more common in the craniofacial region than AVMs; they tend to cause fewer symptoms and less destruction. Managing vascular malformations in the head and neck region presents unique challenges due to the complex anatomy and the critical functions of the structures involved. These malformations can affect vital areas such as the airway, nerves, blood vessels, and muscles, leading to both functional impairments and cosmetic concerns.

History

Symptoms – may be variable

- Onset, timing, and duration
- Laterality
- Progression
- Preceding lesion
- Pain
- Bleeding

Systems

- Airway – aspiration/choking, drooling
- Cardiac – SOB, palpitations, ankle swelling
- Oesophagus – dysphagia, odynophagia
- Voice – dysphonia
- Systemic – symptoms of cardiac failure

DOI: 10.1201/9781003493310-24

Table 22.1 Schobinder's Clinical Staging System

Stage	Description
Stage I (quiescence)	Pink-bluish stain, warmth
Stage II (expansion)	Enlargement, pulsations, thrill, bruit and tense/tortuous veins
Stage III (destruction)	Dystrophic skin changes, ulceration, destruction, tissue necrosis, bleeding or persistent pain
Stage IV (decompensation)	Cardiac failure

Table 22.2 SECg Staging System

Stage		Description
S (surgical/anatomical)	S1	The AVM involves one single anatomical site
	S2	Two adjacent anatomical sites are involved
	S3	Orbital cone, the tongue or the larynx
	S4	Vital structures such as the carotid artery, internal jugular vein and/or base of skull
E (endovascular)	E1	Arteriovenous
	E2	Arteriolovenous
	E3	Arteriolovenuluar
C (clinical features or complications)	C0	No symptoms or complications are present
	C1	Symptomatic without complications – pulsations (or thrills and bruits), paraesthesia, visible swelling
	C2	Local complications – ulceration, infection, haemorrhage
	C3	Systemic complications – congestive cardiac failure
G (growth)	G-	Stable in last 6 months
	G+	Progressive in last 6 months

Past medical history

- Bleeding diatheses
- Cardiovascular history
- Previous malignancy and treatment (especially radiotherapy)

Social history

- Smoking, alcohol status
- Performance status
- Impact on quality of life and occupation, activities of daily living, hobbies
- Impact on psychosocial state – self-esteem, visibility, social interactions, mental health

Family history

- Vascular malformations in family – potential genetic component

Examination

- General inspection – visible asymmetry, deformity
- Assessment of lesion (Figure 22.1)
  - Inspection – size, shape, colour, skin changes, discolouration (red, blue, purple), swelling, visible pulsation, skin breakdown/necrosis
  - Palpation – temperature, pulsation, compressibility and refill, firmness, transillumination
  - Auscultation – bruit, vascular sounds
- Skin – ulceration, discolouration, infection, bleeding, previous trauma
- Functional assessment – neck ROM, muscle of facial expression
- Examine eyes, nose, mouth for functional impairment/distortion

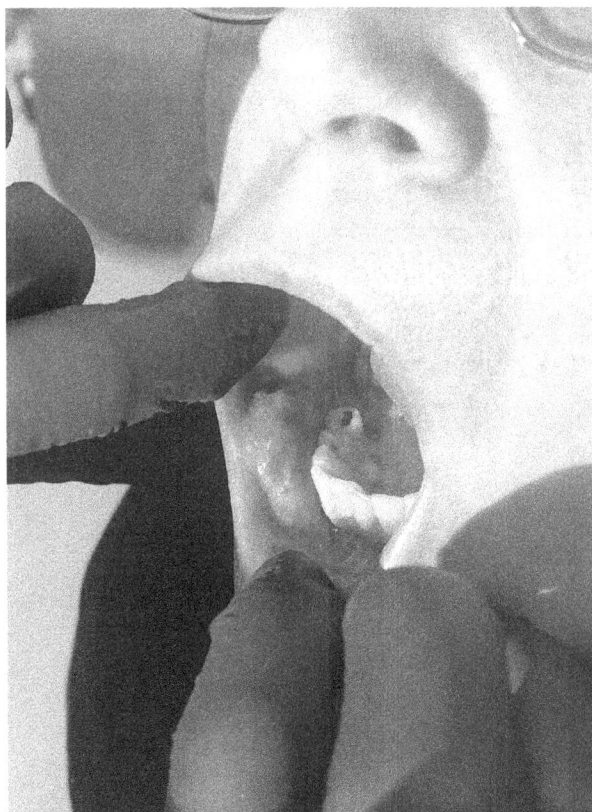

Figure 22.1 Right buccal mucosa vascular tumour.

Signs of a high-flow malformation (AVM)

- Visible pulsation
- Warm
- Lack of compressibility
- Fast refill
- Bruit/vascular sounds
- Local destruction/growth

Management

The principles of management for patients with vascular malformations include reducing or eliminating symptoms such as pain, bleeding, or functional impairments as well as controlling the growth of the malformation and preventing complications. Improving aesthetic outcomes, particularly in visible areas of the face and neck, can often be a cornerstone of management. The management of head and neck vascular malformations is multidisciplinary, often involving specialists from surgery, radiology, dermatology and interventional radiology. The treatment approach is highly individualized and depends on factors such as the type of malformation (high flow vs low flow), its size, location and the symptoms it produces. Management options range from conservative observation in asymptomatic cases to more aggressive interventions like surgery, laser therapy, sclerotherapy or embolization.

Bedside tests

- Bloods and ECG – may be employed for a baseline status

Imaging

- Doppler
- MRI – distinguish different types
- Angiogram

Treatment modalities

- Sclerotherapy
  - Treatment of choice in venous malformation and macrocytic lymphatic malformation
  - Intra-lesion injection of a sclerosing agent induces inflammation, fibrosis, and scarring, causing obliteration and shrinkage of the lymphatic malformation
- Embolization
  - Currently used in combination with surgical resection for AVM
  - Can be used temporarily in cases of major bleeding
- Surgery
  - Complete excision – early-stage, small, localised lesions
  - Surgery and preoperative embolization – high-flow or extensive lesions

Commonly used sclerosants

- Ethanol
- Doxycycline
- Bleomycin
- Sodium tetradecyl sulfate
- OK-432 (Picibanil) – derivative from a killed strain of group A *Streptococcus pyogenes*

Discharge and follow-up

- Follow-up is dependent on the underlying diagnosis and patient factors.
- Most cases require long-term follow-up with active surveillance to assess for recurrence.

MCQs

1) According to the Schobinger clinical staging system, which stage is characterized by tissue necrosis, bleeding and persistent pain?

   A) Stage I (quiescence)
   B) Stage II (expansion)
   C) Stage III (destruction)
   D) Stage IV (decompensation)
   E) Not applicable

2) Which of the following is the treatment of choice for a venous malformation or macrocytic lymphatic malformation?

   A) Surgery
   B) Sclerotherapy
   C) Laser therapy
   D) Systemic steroids
   E) Embolization

3) Which of the following is a hallmark clinical feature of a high-flow vascular malformation (AVM)?

   A) Compressibility and slow refill
   B) Visible pulsation and fast refill
   C) Bluish discolouration and lack of pulsation
   D) Absence of bruit or vascular sounds
   E) Airway compromise

Benign oral lesions
Neha Vatish and Adil Aslam

Background

Benign oral lesions are tissues that have shown a degree of change or abnormality compared to the normal oral mucosa. Importantly, these changes do not show signs of malignancy and can present in the oral cavity in several ways with varying aetiology. While many can occur under conjunction with systemic disease, others are considered idiopathic. Table 23.1 summarises commonly encountered benign oral lesions. It is vital to understand their differing characteristics and differentiate them from pre-malignant and malignant lesions to ensure they are treated appropriately. Management can occur in primary and/or secondary care depending on the extent of the lesion and factors involved. Many benign lesions can self-resolve or require improved oral hygiene and lifestyle changes, whereas others may require further intervention such as surgical removal.

History

Symptoms

- Onset, timing and duration
- Laterality/location
- Preceding events/factors – e.g., trauma
- Growth
- Associated pain/discomfort

Systems

- Oral – difficulty brushing, difficulty chewing, oral hygiene, recent dental infection/treatment
- Oesophagus – dysphagia, odynophagia
- Voice – change in voice
- Systemic – skin involvement, GI symptoms

Past medical history

- Systemic disease – especially autoimmune, dermatological or GI disease
- Previous oral lesion/oral cavity malignancy
- States of immunocompromise

DOI: 10.1201/9781003493310-25

Table 23.1 Different Types of Benign Oral Lesions

Type	Aetiology	Characteristics	Location
Geographic tongue (benign migratory glossitis/erythema migrans)	Unknown Inflammatory	• Atrophic areas of the tongue with a demarcated white border • Rapidly appear then disappear • Depapillated • Lesion and pain can be exacerbated by acidic foods or cheeses	• Dorsum and lateral tongue • Can appear as though moving around the tongue
Hairy tongue	Unknown	• Elongation of the filiform papilla with increased keratin • Pigmentation can occur depending on smoking, diet and oral bacteria • Mostly asymptomatic • Increased risk in smokers, reduced oral hygiene, hyposalivation	• Dorsal tongue
Pseudomembranous candidiasis	Fungal infection	• Creamy plaque on erythematous mucosal base • Can be wiped off easily • Increased risk in immunocompromised patients	• Buccal mucosa, tongue, palate
Erythematous candidiasis	Yeast infection	• Shiny, red lesion • Atrophic and painful • Exacerbated by acidic and spicy foods • Seen in immunocompromised patients and following broad-spectrum antibiotics and steroids	• Tongue, palate
Median rhomboid glossitis	Chronic candida infection	• Symmetrical, well demarcated • Oval/rhomboid shaped • Erythematous, depapillated with a smooth and shiny surface • Increased risk in smoking and steroid use	• Central dorsal tongue

(Continued)

Table 23.1 (Continued)

Type	Aetiology	Characteristics	Location
Lichen planus (non-pre-malignant)	Autoimmune	• Hyperkeratosis • Reticular pattern seen as white striations (Wickham's striae) • Well demarcated • No ulceration or significant erythema	• Bilateral and posterior buccal mucosa but can occur in other areas
Pemphigus vulgaris	Autoimmune	• Intraepithelial blistering of oral mucosa and skin with erosions • Superficial bullae are fluid-filled and easily burst creating ulcerations	• Primary lesions usually affect the palate
Pemphigoid (mucous membrane pemphigoid)	Autoimmune	• Subepithelial blistering of oral mucosa • Red and shiny • Blood-filled bullae can rupture and scar • May have desquamative gingivitis • Increased risk in elderly	• Buccal mucosa, palate, gums
Recurrent aphthous stomatitis (RAS)	Unknown – can indicated systemic involvement	• Oral mucosa ulceration • *Major* – >10 mm, <10 weeks duration, scarring • *Minor* – painful, multiple concomitant ulcers, <10 mm, <2 weeks duration, no scarring • *Herpetiform* – painful, clustered, 2–3 mm, up to 100 ulcers at a time, <2 weeks duration	• Major: keratinised oral mucosa • Minor: non-keratinised mucosa • Herpetiform: keratinised and non-keratinised
Pyogenic granuloma	Unknown/trauma response	• High vascularisation and pedunculated • Rapid growth • Easy bleeding	• Anterior gingiva
Giant cell epulis	Reactive to local irritation	• Red localised swelling • Increased risk in patients with poor oral hygiene	• Gingival or alveolar mucosa
Fibroepithelial polyp	Unknown/trauma response	• Pedunculated or sessile firm growths • Varied size • Usually painless	• Palatal mucosa and other areas

(Continued)

Table 23.1 Different Types of Benign Oral Lesions (Continued)

Type	Aetiology	Characteristics	Location
Frictional keratosis	Repeated trauma	• White textured patches that can be rough • Resolves once trauma removed	• Buccal mucosa, lips, lateral tongue
Mandibular tori	Unknown	• Painless, slow-growing bony growths • Usually bilateral • Flat or spindle-shaped	• Lingually on mandible or hard palate
Papilloma (wart)	HPV infection	Asymptomatic Multiple pink or white papules Slow-growing	Lips, tongue, gums, oropharynx

Social history

- Smoking, alcohol status
- Nutritional status
- Betel nut chewing
- Diet – foods that may cause irritation or exacerbate lesions (e.g., spicy food)
- Oral hygiene status

Allergies

- Allergies to metals in dental restorative materials or other dental products such as toothpaste that can cause or exacerbate lesions
- Drug allergies

Examination

- General inspection – nutritional status, signs of skin or GI disease
- Lesion (Figures 23.1 and 23.2)
  - Site, size, colour, borders, texture
  - Ulceration/induration, erosion
  - Pain
  - Relationship to nearby structures and local tissue
- Oral cavity
  - Extent of lesion
  - Hard and soft palate
  - Altered sensation of lip/tongue
  - Tongue mobility
  - Trismus
- Dental considerations
  - Tooth mobility and dental assessment including occlusion
  - Restorations present in close proximity
  - Oral hygiene
- Neck – regional lymphadenopathy

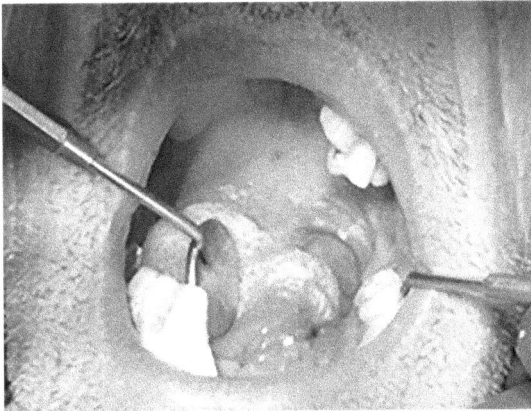

Figure 23.1 Candida infection of the tongue and soft palate.

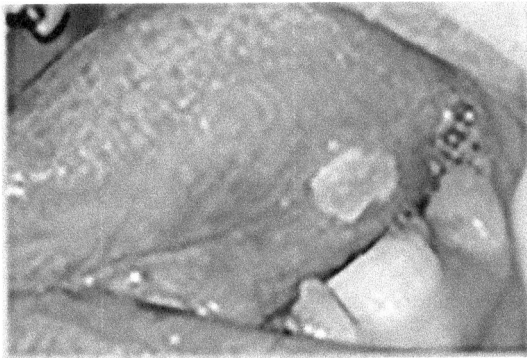

Figure 23.2 Left lateral tongue leukoplakia.

Management

The principle of managing benign oral lesions consists of recording the lesion and undertaking clinical photography to allow accurate monitoring by GDPs. Initial management requires careful examination similar to that of pre-malignant lesions. In addition, the GDP must use this knowledge to see if they can be sufficiently diagnosed and treated within primary care or if a referral to a specialist within secondary care and the MDT is appropriate. Management for each lesion can vary from local measures, dental modifications, medications for systemic or local disease, to surgical removal.

Primary care

- Modify lifestyle factors
  - Smoking cessation
  - Dietary changes
  - Alcohol reduction
  - Mouth rinse after corticosteroid inhaler

- Aim to remove traumatic/irritative factors
  - Adjust dentition – sharp teeth, crowding
- Remove allergens
  - SLS-free toothpaste
  - Nickel within dental appliances
- Identify lesions that are self-resolving and require a watchful wait approach
- Medication – depending on cause
  - Antifungal
  - Chlorhexidine mouthwash
  - Corticosteroids
  - Analgesia
- Review
  - Usually in 1–2 weeks after initial examination of the lesion and removal of potential other causative factors to check for resolution
  - Educate patients to self-monitor lesions and to re-present if changes occur between initial exam and follow-up
  - If regression and improvement is identified, recall patient in 3–6 months with safety netting
  - If no improvement, consider onward referral

When to refer from primary care

- No obvious causative factor can be identified
- Lesion has progressed or changed
- Lesion present for >3 weeks
- High-risk site
- History of pre-malignant lesions
- History of oral cancer

Secondary care

- Lesions can often be further investigated with various options
  - Swabs – mc&s may be useful if infection is suspected
  - Blood tests
    - Anaemia and haematinics – Hb, ferritin, B12, folate (approximately 20% of cases are due to haematological deficiencies)
    - Indirect antibody immunofluorescence in vesiculobullous diseases
  - Excisional/incisional biopsy
  - Incisional biopsies
    - Rule out dysplasia and malignancy in suspicious looking lesions such as frictional keratosis and lichen planus
    - Direct immunofluorescence in suspected vesiculobullous diseases
    - Excisional biopsies are the mainstay for removing small intraoral soft tissue masses
  - Imaging rarely required for benign oral lesions
- Treatment options
  - Medication such as antifungal in suspected fungal infections
  - Excision – laser, cryotherapy, surgery
  - Further treatment for systemic health conditions

- Correction of anaemia and haematological deficiencies
- Dehydration and impaired swallow may require IV hydration/NGT – usually seen in vesiculobullous diseases (such as pemphigus)
- Cutaneous involvement in pemphigus risks significant dehydration and infection risks which can be fatal
  - Early input from dermatology colleagues
  - High-dose prednisolone
    - Pemphigoid – onward referral to ophthalmology (risk of conjunctival scarring and blindness)

MCQs

1) Which of the following lesions typically appears as a result of local irritation as a localised red swelling?

A) Frictional keratosis
B) Mandibular tori
C) Lichen planus
D) Ulcer
E) Giant cell epulis

2) Which of the following lesions is associated with autoimmune disease?

A) Pemphigoid
B) Candida
C) Papilloma
D) Geographic tongue
E) Hairy tongue

3) Which blood test can form an important investigation for benign oral lesions?

A) Urea
B) Creatinine
C) Calcium
D) Ferritin
E) Magnesium

Chapter 24

Pre-malignant oral lesions

Neha Vatish and Adil Aslam

Background

Pre-malignant lesions are characterised as lesions with a greater risk of abnormal cell transformation rate within the oral and surrounding mucosa, that therefore have the potential to result in a cancerous lesion. Although approximately less than 5% of the world population are affected by oral pre-cancerous lesions, they contribute up to 35% of diagnosed oral malignancies with a greater incidence identified in males. A vast number of external factors such as tobacco and alcohol intake as well as local and systemic influences including HPV and candida infections can further increase the malignancy risk. It is vital to recognise their differing characteristics to monitor changes and determine the appropriate course of action.

History

Symptoms

- Onset, timing and duration
- Laterality/location
- Preceding events/factors – e.g., different lesion
- Growth
- Associated pain/discomfort

Systems

- Oral – difficulty brushing, difficulty chewing, oral hygiene, recent dental infection/treatment
- Oesophagus – dysphagia, odynophagia
- Voice – change in voice
- Systemic – skin involvement, GI symptoms

Past medical history

- Systemic disease – especially autoimmune, dermatological or GI disease
- Previous oral lesion/oral cavity malignancy
- States of immunocompromise

DOI: 10.1201/9781003493310-26

Table 24.1 Different Types of Pre-Malignant Oral Lesions

Lesion	Characteristics
Leukoplakia	• White patch in the oral mucosa • Most common subtypes are homogenous and non-homogenous • Cannot be attributed to any other lesion or disease *Homogenous* • Plaque-like lesions • Uniform smooth or wrinkled surface • Less risk of transforming into malignancy *Non-homogenous* • Speckled varied appearance with increased keratin • Less circumscribed • Nodules and ulceration may occur • Common as multifocal lesions • Increased risk of malignant transformation
Erythroplakia	• Red, velvety and smooth patches with well-demarcated borders • Solitary • High-risk sites of oral mucosa • High risk of malignant changes • Cannot be attributed to any other lesion or disease
Erythroleukoplakia (speckled leukoplakia)	• Combined red and white patches • High risk of malignant change
Submucous fibrosis	• Chronic and progressive oral connective tissue scarring • Pale mucosa with fibrous banding • Associated with trismus and lip and cheek immobility • Increased risk with betel nut chewing
Candida leucoplakia (chronic hyperplastic candidiasis)	• White patch • Seen bilaterally on oral commissural buccal mucosa or tongue dorsum • Increased risk in male heavy smokers
Erosive lichen planus	• Variant of oral lichen planus • Painful and chronic ulcerations of the oral mucosa • Glazed, red lesions with defined borders and scarring • Wickham's striae may be seen • Pain can affect eating habits

Social history

- Smoking, alcohol status
- Betel nut chewing
- Nutritional status
- Diet – foods that may cause irritation or exacerbate lesions (e.g., spicy food)
- Oral hygiene status

Examination

- General inspection – nutritional status, signs of skin or GI disease
- Lesion (Figure 24.1)
  - Site, size, colour, borders, texture
  - Ulceration/erosion
  - Induration
  - Pain
  - Relationship to nearby structures and local tissue
- Oral cavity
  - Extent of lesion
  - Hard and soft palate
  - Altered sensation of lip/tongue
  - Tongue mobility
  - Trismus
  - Tooth mobility and dental assessment
- Neck – regional lymphadenopathy

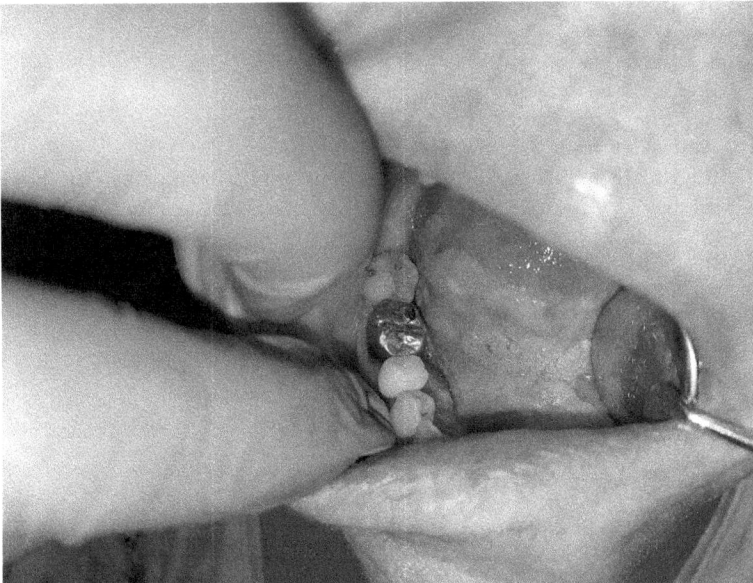

Figure 24.1 Proliferative verrucous leukoplakia (PVL) and alveolar SCC of the right oral cavity.

High-risk sites for oral cavity malignancy

- Floor of the mouth
- Ventral surface and lateral borders of the tongue
- Retromolar pad
- Soft palate
- Palatine tonsils
- Areas in contact with habitual behaviours (e.g., buccal mucosa exposed to betel nut poses a greater risk of buccal leukoplakia and malignant transformation)

Management

The principle of managing pre-malignant oral lesions involves early identification and appropriate monitoring or treatment depending on the lesion type. Initial management begins during an examination by a GDP in primary care. Accurate documentation of the lesion is vital for short- and long-term management. Clinical photographs are advised to assist in monitoring changes. For short-term management, when appropriate, the elimination of potential causative factors can allow for the lesion to be assessed and resolved, and aetiology identified. This process is required to determine if the lesion is actually pre-malignant or if it forms part of a differential diagnosis including frictional keratosis, lichen planus or a lichenoid reaction. From this GDPs are able to assess if a patient requires a referral to a specialist and MDT within secondary care for further investigations and treatment.

Primary care

- Onward referral to secondary care if pre-malignant lesions are highly suspected
- Modify lifestyle factors
  - Smoking cessation
  - Dietary changes
  - Alcohol reduction
  - Mouth rinse after corticosteroid inhaler
- Aim to remove traumatic/irritative factors
  - Adjust dentition – sharp teeth, crowding
- If it is unclear whether the lesion is pre-malignant then the patient can be reviewed in 1–2 weeks following removal of potential other causative factors

When to refer from primary care

- No obvious causative factor can be identified
- Lesion has progressed or changed
- Lesion present for >3 weeks
- High-risk site
- History of pre-malignant lesions
- History of oral cancer

Secondary care

- Lesions can often be further investigated and treated with various options
  - Incisional biopsy
    - Mainstay practice in secondary care to rule out dysplasia and malignancy
    - Mild dysplasia often requires risk factor modification and surveillance
    - Moderate or severe dysplasia usually results in excision of the lesion
    - Biopsies should be representative of the lesion as a whole
  - Antifungal therapy in candidal leukoplakia
    - Confirm with biopsy
    - Systemic antifungals (e.g., fluconazole)
    - May require re-biopsy following antifungal to differentiate reactive cellular atypia from genuine dysplasia
  - Blood tests and cross-sectional imaging are not usually required unless malignancy is suspected
  - Ongoing surveillance programme with emphasis on risk factor reduction and a low threshold to repeat incisional biopsies as required

MCQs

1) Which of the following lesions is typically described as red, velvety and smooth patches with well-demarcated borders?

   A) Leukoplakia
   B) Erythroplakia
   C) Erythroleukoplakia
   D) Lichen planus
   E) Lichen sclerosus

2) Which of the following lesions can be associated with trismus?

   A) Leukoplakia
   B) Erythroplakia
   C) Candida leukoplakia
   D) Submucous fibrosis
   E) Lichen planus

3) Which is not a high-risk site for oral cavity malignancy?

   A) Floor of the mouth
   B) Ventral surface and lateral borders of the tongue
   C) Retromolar pad
   D) Soft palate
   E) Hard palate

Section III

MCQ Answers and Explanations

Chapter 1: Odontogenic infections

1) C
2) C
3) C

Explanations

1) Although IV antibiotics are included in the management of this patient the first port of call is to ensure that the airway is not critical due to the presenting symptom of neck swelling and dysphagia. Bloods and lactate can be done as part of the investigations but do not take precedence over the airway.
2) Here there is no immediate airway threat. The patient needs incision and drainage of the abscess and extraction of the tooth, which will give the best management. Since the swelling is localised and intraoral, extraoral drainage is not warranted. Discharge is not appropriate because the infection can further spread if not treated timely.
3) The patient is talking in clear sentences and can swallow; therefore, there is no immediate airway concern. He will ultimately need incision and drainage but this is not an emergency that needs to be performed overnight, and so he can be managed medically until the procedure can be performed during daylight hours. Extraoral drainage should not be performed in the ED.

Chapter 2: Osteomyelitis

1) B
2) C
3) C

Explanations

1) Mandibular osteomyelitis most commonly arises from the direct spread of infection associated with necrotic pulp, periodontal disease, or inadequate dental treatment. While haematogenous spread and radiation exposure are possible causes, they are less common.
2) Garre osteomyelitis is characterized by periosteal bone formation, often described as an "onion-skin" appearance on radiographs. This condition usually arises from long-standing, low-grade dentoalveolar infections, particularly in younger patients.
3) Sequestrectomy and saucerization are the first-line surgical treatments for chronic suppurative osteomyelitis, aiming to remove non-viable bone and promote healing. Decortication is also commonly used in more chronic or extensive cases.

Chapter 3: Ludwig's angina, necrotising fasciitis and airway compromise

1) B
2) A
3) C

Explanations

1) This patient needs immediate airway management with anaesthetic support. The patient will not be able to lie flat for CT and it can further compromise his airway. Transferring to theatre will require some time and is not the correct option in this scenario. Stepwise airway management with intubation should be preferred. Incision and drainage are needed, but only after the airway is secured. IV antibiotics form a part of the management plan, but again, airway management comes first.

2) This patient requires an urgent scan to assess for further collection. There is no airway issue and at day 3 there is no indication of tracheostomy tube change. At this hour, and if the airway is secure there is no need for an urgent surgical intervention. The antibiotics might need to be changed or escalated by adding further antibiotics in conjunction with microbiology but only after further information is gathered from imaging.

3) Surgical drainage and debridement of necrotic tissue is the primary goal in management of necrotising fasciitis in patients with no immediate airway threat. IV antibiotics and fluid are a part of management, but not the primary goal. Skin grafting on an infected bed is not ideal.

Chapter 4: Osteonecrosis of the jaw

1) C
2) D
3) A

Explanations

1) MRONJ specifically excludes patients with a history of radiation therapy to the jaw or metastatic disease. While the other options are associated with MRONJ, radiation therapy to the jaw is a risk factor for ORN, not MRONJ.

2) Stage II MRONJ involves exposed necrotic bone, associated pain, and infection or purulence. Stage I includes exposed bone without infection, Stage III involves advanced infection with complications like fractures, and Stage 0 has no exposed bone but presents with unexplained symptoms like pain.

3) Bisphosphonates bind to bone hydroxyapatite, inhibiting osteoclast activity and reducing bone turnover. This can impair the natural healing processes of the bone, especially after trauma or invasive dental procedures, increasing the risk of MRONJ.

Chapter 5: Mandibular trauma

1) C
2) B
3) E

Explanations

1) The inferior alveolar nerve travels through the ramus and body of the mandible exiting at the mental foramen. It can be injured during a fracture of the mandibular angle.

2) A displaced fracture in the tooth-bearing section of the mandible is classified as an open fracture and requires prophylactic antibiotics. Undisplaced mandibular fractures are often managed conservatively and an open approach to a mandibular condyle fracture often is carried out by a trans-parotid approach and may cause weakness of the facial nerve because it traverses through the parotid gland.

3) RTAs were previously the most common cause of a fractured mandible, but since widespread use of seatbelts, this is no longer the case. Fractured mandibles now occur most commonly due to interpersonal trauma.

Chapter 6: Midface trauma

1) B
2) B
3) D

Explanations

1) The inferior rectus attaches to the inferior aspect of the globe. In orbital floor fractures this muscle may herniate through the fracture or become entrapped by the bony fragments causing restriction of upward gaze and double vision.

2) Zygomatic complex fractures often fracture in one or more locations including the orbital rim, zygomatic arch and at the zygomatic buttress. The infraorbital nerve which supplies the cheek is often affected during these injuries and the patient may present with paraesthesia. Le Fort fractures may present with a malocclusion and mobility of the maxilla, and isolated orbital floor fractures may present with numbness of the cheek but often have subconjunctival haemorrhage and diplopia.

3) This scenario describes a retrobulbar haemorrhage occurring postoperatively. This is an emergency and requires urgent evacuation of the haematoma and control of the bleeding. Given that the patient is postop and in recovery, the best course would be for an immediate return to theatre.

Chapter 7: Orbital trauma

1) B
2) C
3) B

Explanations

1) This is a sight-threatening emergency caused by bleeding behind the eye, leading to increased intraorbital pressure.

2) Coronal formatting of non-contrast (bone window) CT is the modality of choice to diagnose orbital fractures. It is also used in surgical planning in patient-specific orbital wall implants.

3) White eye syndrome, caused by the oculocardiac reflex, may be misinterpreted by clinicians as a sign of head injury. It requires prompt intervention to avoid long-term complications.

Chapter 8: Frontal bone trauma

1) B
2) D
3) A

Explanations

1) Whilst all of these might be present with an underlying frontal fracture, the most significant injury would be a posterior wall fracture with dural tear, which would most likely present as CSF rhinorrhoea.
2) Cosmesis is the only common indication for anterior wall repair. Dural tear, outflow tract obstruction and brow ptosis are unlikely to be associated with an isolated anterior wall fracture. The risk of supraorbital paraesthesia may be increased by surgical intervention.
3) Exposing the cribriform plate requires stripping of the olfactory nerves and creates anosmia and requires a lot of frontal lobe retraction. Cribriform fractures with CSF leakage are normally treated with transnasal obstruction procedures. The other steps are key to successful cranialisation and obstruction of nasofrontal outflow tracts.

Chapter 9: Facial ballistic trauma

1) C
2) B
3) E

Explanations

1) The energy deposited into tissues by the projectile is the most important determinant of injury severity because it reflects the damage caused by the projectile's interaction with the surrounding structures. While velocity, firearm type and distance contribute to this energy, they are secondary factors compared to the direct impact of energy transfer.
2) Immediate surgical exploration is warranted in cases of airway or circulatory compromise because these are life-threatening emergencies. While other factors such as soft tissue injury, imaging availability, or fractures are important, they do not outweigh the need to prioritize airway and circulation in the decision-making process.
3) Free flap surgery is often used to reconstruct complex defects, ensuring functional and aesthetic rehabilitation.

Chapter 10: Soft tissue injuries

1) B
2) C
3) A

Explanations

1) Bloods, past medical history and prior medications are all important information. However, a trauma CT will alert you to other injuries this patient may

have sustained which may affect your management plan (may be too unwell for repair under local anaesthesia, immobilisation due to C-spine injuries etc.). Mechanism of injury was significant (driver died on scene). Rushing to the patient without adequate information may cause more harm than good.

2) Deep layers should be repaired first – failure to do so will result in functional problems (uneven movement of muscles when smiling). Aesthetically, how the vermillion border meets will be the most important surgical factor. Early local anaesthesia infiltration (especially with epinephrine) will cause blanching and swelling of tissues. This will result in uneven tissue distribution and will make the vermillion border look less obvious. For closure of skin on the lip, use non-dissolvable sutures for dry vermillion and dissolvable for wet vermillion for best aesthetic outcome. In non-compliant patients (paediatric, learning difficulties), dissolvable sutures throughout may be more appropriate.

3) Provided the forehead laceration does not extend down to muscle, adjuncts can be used to close the wound. This is especially useful in the paediatric patient who may not tolerate local anaesthesia, and it will avoid general anaesthesia. Cat bite wounds should always be washed and explored (they tend to be deeper than they look!). Aesthetically, lip lacerations crossing the vermillion border should be repaired with sutures for the best outcome. Soft tissue injury on any facial organ (nose, eyes, ears, lips) should be repaired with sutures when possible due to the complex 3D topography of these structures. Abrasions often don't need tension closure (unless planned for excision and closure of abrasion for cosmetic purposes).

Chapter 11: TMJ dislocation

1) A
2) C
3) A

Explanations

1) TMJ dislocation is most commonly anterior. Posterior, superior or lateral dislocation is rarer and may be associated with fractures or trauma to adjacent structures.
2) The bimanual method is the most commonly used method for closed reductions in TMJ dislocation. The external and gag methods are reasonable alternatives. Botulinum toxin and intra-articular injections are not appropriate for closed reductions.
3) Circumferential chin bandage is most appropriate following reduction. Most patients do not require IMF or nasogastric feeding. Tracheostomy and pro-longed inpatient stay are not appropriate.

Chapter 12: Neck haematoma

1) D
2) C
3) D

Explanations

1) Neck haematoma is usually caused by generalised ooze of blood or slippage of ligature. It is prudent to achieve sound haemostasis and ligation of potential bleeding vessels. Meticulous surgery, attention to detail, and performing a head-down Valsalva at the end of the operation can help to prevent neck haematoma, potential threat to airway, return to theatre, and patient morbidity.
2) Neck haematoma could be stable or expanding due to slow ooze of blood in a closed neck compartment, especially in patients with no tracheostomy. This is a surgical emergency because it could lead to compression of airway, airway oedema, and subsequent risk to life. The airway should be assessed and secured promptly.
3) Expanding neck haematoma poses risk to airway, blood loss, and compression of neurovascular structures. Once the airway is secured, expanding neck haematoma needs prompt exploration and assessment of neck vessels with the aim of identifying and securing bleeding vessels followed by evacuation of clots and neck washout. This also helps to improve healing by preventing postoperative neck infection.

Chapter 13: Free flap compromise

1) D
2) C
3) C
4) B
5) B

Explanations

1) Free flap reconstruction of an oro-facial defect provides robust reconstruction which can be matched three dimensionally to the defect allowing functional rehabilitation along with the added advantage of a flap with its own blood supply able to withstand future adjuvant treatment such as radiotherapy.
2) The primary aim of reconstruction of an oral cavity defect is to minimise adverse effects on functions such as speech and swallowing, maintaining tissue forms while minimising cosmetic deformity. Secondary aims of reconstruction are to minimise or prevent scarring and to improve lip seal depending on tissue subunits involved in ablative surgery.
3) Free flaps are mostly prone to venous failure. The first sign of venous compromise is brisk capillary refill, which represents good arterial inflow but sluggish venous drainage. This can progress to a bluish tinge of the flap tissue and later rigidity or firmness of the flap, and consequently flap failure if not timely identified.
4) A pale free flap with no Doppler signal suggests possible poor arterial inflow, hence the need for prompt assessment (some clinicians will do a scratch test to assess blood oozing from the skin/dermal plexus) and return to theatre for assessment of vessel anastomosis.
5) Postoperative timely clinical assessment (flap colour, capillary refill, tissue turgor, Doppler signal, scratch test) with established protocol remains the gold standard for free flap monitoring. Junior doctors or specialist nurses usually carry out these observations and are trained to monitor flaps.

Chapter 14: Oral cavity malignancy

1) A
2) E
3) D

Explanations

1) A persistent non-healing ulcer present for >3 weeks is a common presentation and should be urgently referred on a 2-week wait pathway. Change in voice and a neck lump can be more suggestive of malignancies of the upper aerodigestive tract. Restricted range of neck motion and trismus are non-specific in this context.
2) Surgery is generally considered the primary treatment modality for oral cavity malignancy. Radiotherapy is commonly used in the adjuvant setting and may also be considered in those unfit for surgery.
3) A minimum of 5 years of clinical surveillance is recommended. Many patients do, however, continue annual surveillance after this point.

Chapter 15: Cutaneous malignancy

1) B
2) C
3) E

Explanations

1) According to the BAD guidance this is a high-risk SCC of the ear. He is young and therefore primary RT should not be offered; it also carries additional risks of radionecrosis. The correct answer would be to excise with a 6 mm margin.
2) According to the BAD guidance, this is classified as a high-risk SCC based on the degree of differentiation and the ear is a high-risk site. Therefore, the follow-up should be 2 years.
3) This is likely to be a cutaneous melanoma. However, it is not clear if the entire lesion is melanoma or if there is a focus of melanoma surrounded by lentigo maligna (melanoma in situ). You should never excise a suspected melanoma with a wide excision prior to biopsy. Radiotherapy has no role in curative strategies in melanoma, particularly without tissue diagnosis. Excision with a 2 mm margin may be an option; however, this carries significant morbidity if there is in fact only a small focus of melanoma. Therefore, mapping biopsies with a clearly labelled photo is the best course of action.

Chapter 16: Salivary gland disease

1) B
2) B
3) B

Explanations

1) A salivary gland stone, most commonly affecting the submandibular gland specifically, is the most common cause of obstructive sialadenitis. Management

depends on the location of the stone with the duct, the size of the stone, and the patient's symptoms.

2) Adjuvant radiotherapy is indicated for tumours larger than 4 cm, those with close or positive surgical margins, perineural invasion, multiple metastatic neck nodes, and high-grade adenoid cystic carcinoma.

3) Sialendoscopy is indicated for small stones located within the gland's duct. Most of the glands will resume normal function once the stones are removed.

Chapter 17: Head and neck reconstruction (free flaps)

1) D
2) B
3) A

Explanations

1) Free fibula flaps remain the gold standard for mandibular reconstruction. They provide ample bone for full mandibular reconstruction and restoration of facial form and contour, and provide cortical and cancellous bone that can receive dental implants, which is helpful in functional rehabilitation.

2) Donor site morbidity remains a key challenge in free flap reconstruction. Donor site healing, skin graft failure, nerve function compromise, haematoma, and infection often add to the patient's morbidity and postoperative recovery.

3) The main advantage of free flap reconstruction surgery is its versatility and pro-vision of soft and/or hard tissue, independent of recipient site, with excellent ability to restore surgical defects in all three dimensions. This gives patients the best chance of minimising function and cosmetic deficit that is common follow-ing ablative surgery for tumour resections.

Chapter 18: Orthognathic surgery

1) E
2) E
3) D

Explanations

1) The most likely cause of bleeding in this situation is venous in nature from the pterygoid venous plexus. As with any venous bleeding, applying pressure is the first-line measure. All the options would take time to reduce bleeding. Reducing the blood pressure further with the patient already under hypotensive anaes-thesia can be dangerous and risk a stroke as well as having little direct effect on venous bleeding.

2) This patient is displaying multiple features of body dysmorphic disorder. Although his concerns may be valid, he appears to have taken these beyond context and attributed his difficulties in work to his physical appearance. He is best managed in an MDT setting in which multiple professionals can give their opinions, particularly with a psychologist to help broach this sensitive issue.

3) Relapse of the mandible does not occur intraoperatively. In its earliest form this can occur in the first six weeks postoperatively. This is unlikely to be an unfa-vourable split on one side of the mandible because this would typically result

in displacement of the mandible to the affected side. Fixation failure on both sides of the mandible intraoperatively would be extremely unlikely. Insufficient release of the soft tissue envelope typically results in backwards displacement of the mandible. Incorrect condylar positioning typically occurs in large maxillary impactions when interferences have not sufficiently been trimmed. The condyles have been distracted from the glenoid fossa and this has been translated into the final position.

Chapter 19: TMJ disorders

1) C
2) C
3) C

Explanations

1) Temporalis muscle hyperplasia is not an indication for TMJ replacement. The common indications include rheumatoid arthritis, severe trauma, ankylosis, and osteoarthritis.
2) MRI is preferred for assessing soft tissues like the articular disc and capsule.
3) Nickel is the most commonly presenting component for allergic response.

Chapter 20: TMJ ankylosis

1) C
2) D
3) B

Explanations

1) Trauma to the mandible is a leading cause of TMJ ankylosis.
2) CT scan is the most effective imaging modality for visualizing bony fusion in TMJ ankylosis.
3) Gap arthroplasty is often required to remove the ankylosed portion of the joint followed by TMJ reconstruction either as a single-stage or second-stage procedure.

Chapter 21: Cleft lip and palate

1) C
2) D
3) B

Explanations

1) A hearing test is conducted through the NHSP. This should occur in all neonates soon after birth and is not specific to children with cleft. Lip repairs are usually conducted between 3 and 6 months and palate repairs typically between 6 and 9 months.
2) The Sommerlad repair is a recognised surgery in the UK for secondary palate repair surgery. The vomerine flap closure, Fisher and Millard repairs are options in primary surgery. The Le Fort osteotomy is a type of surgery involved in orthognathic surgery.

3) Whereas a specialist feeding bottle is normally needed to help a cleft child feed, nasogastric or other feeding tubes are not usually required. Tracheostomy indications remain broadly the same for cleft and non-cleft children and hearing rehabilitation is only required if there are confirmed issues with the child's hearing.

Chapter 22: Vascular malformation

1) C
2) B
3) B

Explanations

1) Dystrophic skin changes, ulceration, destruction, tissue necrosis, bleeding or persistent pain are signs of Stage 3.
2) Intra-lesion injection of a sclerosing agent induces inflammation, fibrosis, and scarring, causing obliteration and shrinkage of the lymphatic malformation.
3) Visible pulsation and fast refill: high-flow vascular malformations are locally aggressive lesions that behave clinically as low-grade neoplasms.

Chapter 23: Benign oral lesions

1) E
2) A
3) D

Explanations

1) From all of the listed options, giant cell epulis is typically as a result of local irritation and presents as a localised red swelling. Pyogenic granulomas are also red swellings that present following trauma but these are more commonly found on the anterior gingiva and are not listed as one of the options.
2) Pemphigoid (mucous membrane pemphigoid) has an autoimmune aetiology.
3) Ferriting may be an important investigation to conduct since up to 20% of benign oral lesions are due to haematological deficiencies.

Chapter 24: Pre-malignant oral lesions

1) B
2) D
3) E

Explanations

1) Erythyroplakia is typically described as red, velvety, smooth patches with well-demarcated borders.
2) Submucous fibrosis can be associated with trismus as well as lip and cheek immobility.
3) The hard palate is not deemed a high-risk site for oral cavity malignancy compared to the other options.

Index

Note: Page numbers in *italics* indicate a figure and page numbers in **bold** indicate a table on the corresponding page.

For Product Safety Concerns and Information please contact our EU
representative GPSR@taylorandfrancis.com
Taylor & Francis Verlag GmbH, Kaufingerstraße 24, 80331 München, Germany

www.ingramcontent.com/pod-product-compliance
Lightning Source LLC
Chambersburg PA
CBHW070722220326
41598CB00024BA/3265